The 30-Minute Type 2 Diabetes Cookbook

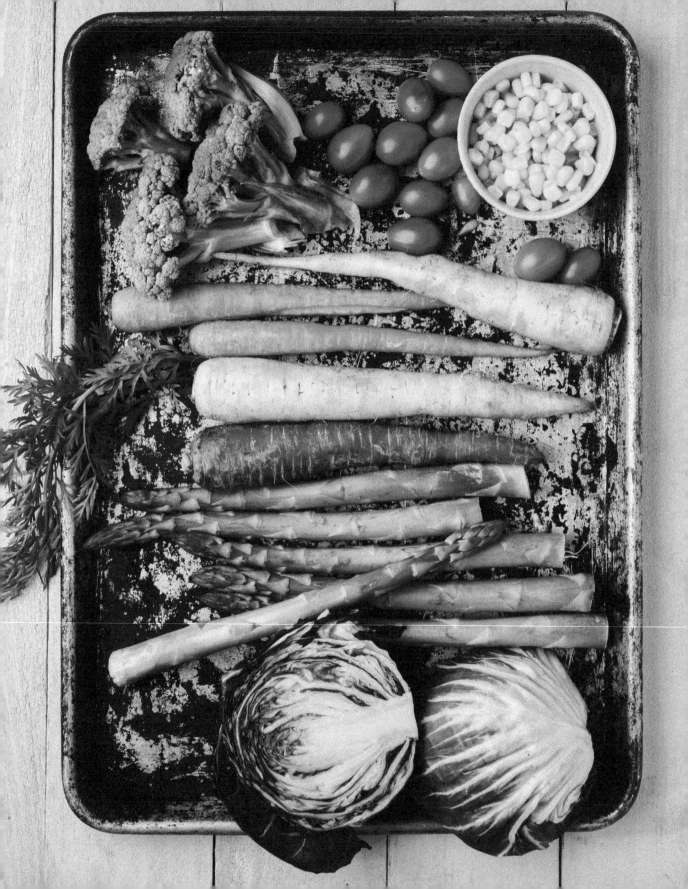

THE 30-MINUTE TYPE 2 DIABETES Cookbook

75 Fuss-Free Recipes for Healthy Eating

Andy De Santis, RD, MPH
Michelle Anderson

ROCKRIDGE PRESS

Interior and Cover Designer: Jami Spittler
Art Producer: Tom Hood
Editor: Anne Lowrey
Production Editor: Ellina Litmanovich
Production Manager: Sandy Noman

Photography © Hélène Dujardin, 2020, cover and pp v; Thomas Story, p. ii; Nadine Greeff, p vi; Andrew Purcell, pp viii and 132; Monika Ross/Stockfood, p. xii; Daxiao Productions/Stocksy, p. 26; Simone Neufing/Stockfood, p. 42; Cameron Whitman/Stocksy, p. 60; Ivan Solis/Stocksy, p. 82; PhotoCuisine/Tom Swalens/Stockfood, p. 102; The Picture Pantry/Stockfood, p. 118. Food styling by Anna Hampton, cover and pp v; Carrie Purcell, p. 132. Author photograph courtesy of Natalie CD Photography.

Paperback ISBN: 978-1-63807-477-9
eBook ISBN: 978-1-63878-238-4
R0

I dedicate this book
to my sister and her new
fiancé, Will. As fellow health
professionals, you
both inspire me to be the
best dietitian I can.
Congratulations
to you both!

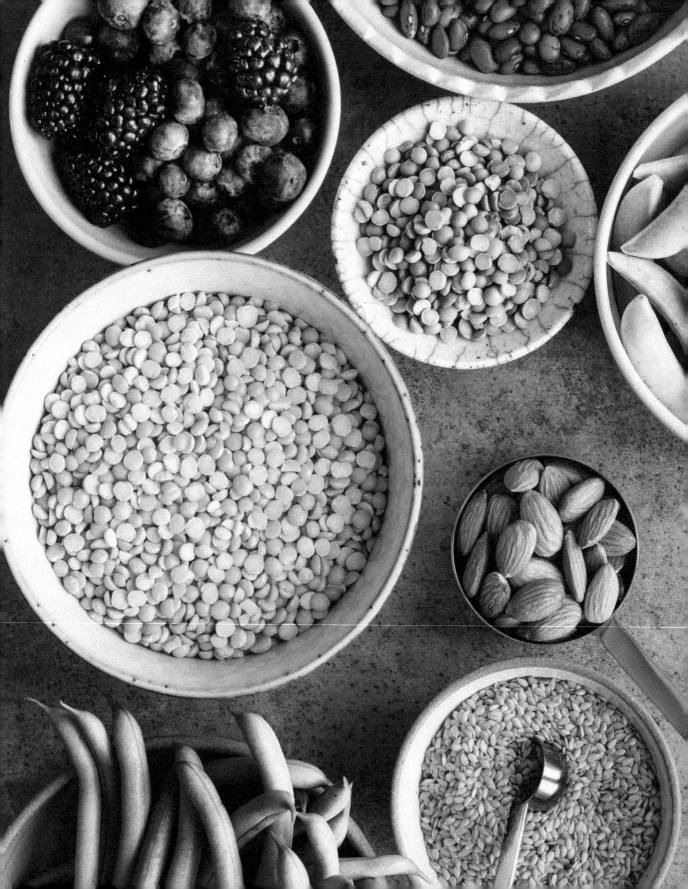

Contents

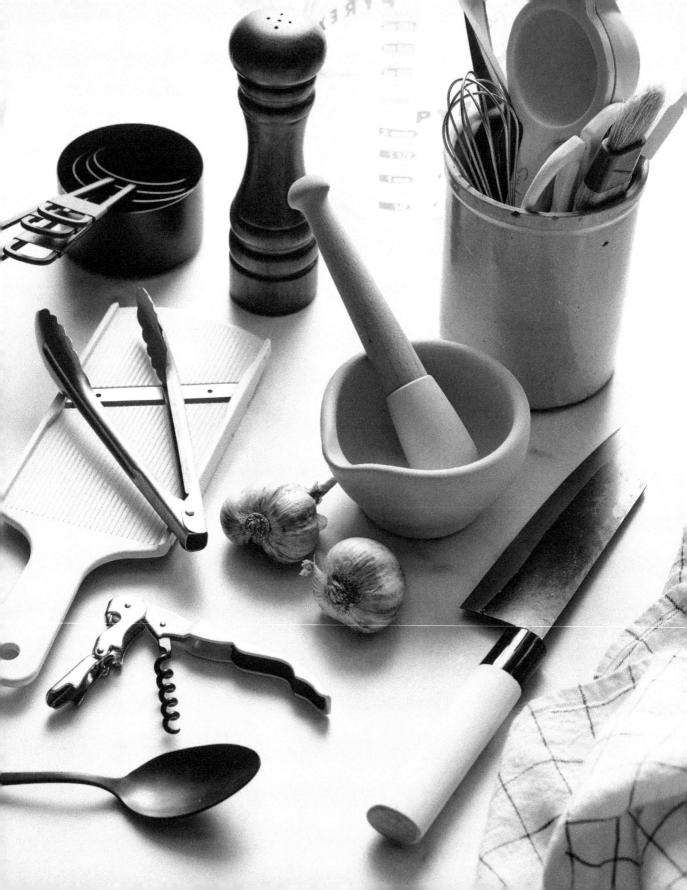

Introduction

Hello everyone! My name is Andy De Santis, and I'm truly thrilled to be your guide on the path toward healthier eating for type 2 diabetes. I'm a private practice dietitian from Toronto, Canada, who has helped many people in your position. Although I am now self-employed, my first job after obtaining my master's degree from the University of Toronto was at the Canadian Diabetes Association (now Diabetes Canada). I spent a good deal of time there working in tandem with very bright scientific minds in this field, and I can appreciate more than most that being newly diagnosed with type 2 diabetes can be daunting.

It's quite possible that you are reading this passage on the heels of a recent type 2 diagnosis and perhaps are a bit scared or uncertain of what is ahead. I want you to know that you are in good hands. My goal with this book is to provide you with the best support and guidance possible as a complement to the care you are receiving from your health care team.

We have nutrition science on our side and so many dietary strategies and tools at our disposal. We'll work to get your blood sugar levels to a better place, reduce your risk of diabetes-related health complications, and, in doing so, help you enjoy a great quality of life going forward.

One of the sayings that used to circulate at Diabetes Canada during my time there was: "The complications of well-controlled diabetes are nothing." This is actually a well-known expression in the world of diabetes care. It essentially means that you, as an individual who has been newly diagnosed with type 2 diabetes, are not relegated to accept the health-related complications that many people associate with diabetes. Together, and in collaboration with your health care team, we can work toward flipping the script on type 2 diabetes and putting you back in the driver's seat of your own health.

I've helped hundreds of clients with newly diagnosed type 2 diabetes utilize the power of nutrition. In chapter 1, I will teach you the very same powerful nutrition science fundamentals that I use with them. From there, my fellow Canadian and the book's recipe developer, chef extraordinaire Michelle Anderson, will show you that eating well with diabetes can be more delicious than you ever imagined. Michelle and I have worked very closely to ensure that the 30-minute creations in our book are fully optimized for your success and in accordance with the appropriate nutrition science principles.

As you go through chapter 1, you will gain a practical understanding of what these important principles are. In the multiple recipe-focused chapters that follow, you will see these principles brought to life. I think you will be pleasantly surprised to see many commonly enjoyed foods and ingredients being utilized because, contrary to what you may have heard, you don't need to follow an overly complex or restrictive diet to achieve good health with type 2 diabetes.

Does all of this sound too good to be true? I invite you to keep reading.

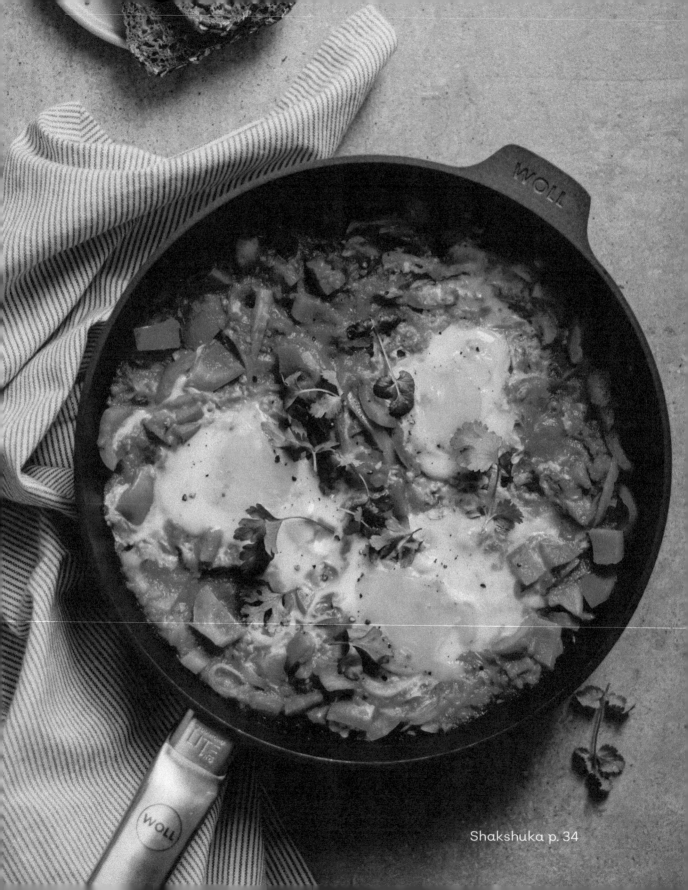

Shakshuka p. 34

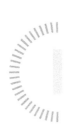

A NEW WAY OF EATING MADE EASY

So, you're newly diagnosed with type 2 diabetes. What happens next? My goal with the first chapter of the book is to begin to answer this question from the dietary perspective.

It's likely you've already received guidance from your health care team, and I'd like you to think of what's written here as a source of further support. Many people I work with who are newly diagnosed with type 2 diabetes operate under the assumption that their diet going forward must be bland, lifeless, and devoid of many of their favorite food groups.

While there are dietary changes that will need to be made for blood sugar control, nutrition for diabetes management does not need to be as restrictive as some people make it out to be. Let's begin with the basics.

An Introduction to Diabetes Nutrition

Recent CDC statistics suggest that around 1 in 10 Americans, amounting to over 34 million people, are currently living with diabetes. The vast majority of these people are living with type 2, with over a million new cases diagnosed annually.

There is also an even larger number of Americans, close to 90 million, living with what is known as prediabetes. A prediabetes diagnosis essentially means that your body is showing signs that it may no longer be properly able to control its blood sugar levels but that the severity is not sufficient to warrant a clinical type 2 diabetes diagnosis. If those living with prediabetes do not make some measure of dietary and/or lifestyle changes, they will end up at higher risk of progressing to type 2 in the future.

The good news is that the guidance, education, and culinary support provided in this book are also fully suitable for anyone living with prediabetes who wants to take control of their blood sugar levels and avoid ultimately ending up with type 2. I'm now going to explain some key terms that we need to carry the conversation forward.

Blood Sugar/Blood Glucose and Insulin

Sugar, in the form of glucose, naturally flows through the human bloodstream within specific ranges that our body tries very hard to maintain. Even so, blood sugar levels can indeed fluctuate due to a number of factors, including our dietary choices in both the short (i.e., right after a meal) and long term (i.e., overall dietary choices). Generally, these ranges are tightly controlled in part by an optimally functioning pancreas that releases the right amount of insulin at the right time and bodily cells that respond to this insulin in a healthy way.

Insulin is the hormone that acts as a sort of key and "opens" your cells to allow glucose from the bloodstream to enter for use as energy and/or storage. The hormone itself was discovered in 1921 by Canadian scientists Frederick Banting and Charles Best at the University of Toronto (the same place where I happened to do my graduate studies in public health nutrition). In people living with type 2 diabetes, various bodily cells may not respond to insulin as well as they used to.

This phenomenon is known as insulin resistance, which essentially means that cells become less responsive to insulin. Thus, the body's ability to allow sugar to enter the cells is compromised, and glucose instead accumulates in the bloodstream. This is a big reason why type 2 diabetes is characterized by higher-than-normal blood sugar levels via a fasting blood glucose or A1C test.

BLOOD SUGAR RANGES*

RESULT**	A1C TEST	FASTING BLOOD SUGAR TEST	RANDOM BLOOD SUGAR TEST
DIABETES	6.5% or above	126 mg/dL or above	200 mg/dL or above
PREDIABETES	5.7 – 6.4%	100 – 125 mg/dL	N/A
NORMAL	Below 5.7%	99 mg/dL or below	N/A

* This table comes from CDC.gov/diabetes/basics/getting-tested.html.
** Only a doctor can diagnose diabetes based on blood work and contextual factors may be considered before a final decision is made.

A1C is essentially a measurement of your average blood sugar levels over a three-month period and is often expressed as a percentage. Your doctor may have diagnosed your diabetes based on your fasting blood glucose, A1C, or both.

Why are high blood sugar levels problematic? Excessive sugar in the blood can damage the more sensitive organs in the body, including the eyes, kidneys, sexual organs, and heart. This explains why chronic poorly managed diabetes greatly increases the risk of issues with these organs, such as heart and kidney disease, among other concerns.

The good news is that the complications associated with well-controlled diabetes are few and far between, and through improved dietary practices, you can improve how your cells respond to insulin and take back control of your blood sugar levels.

Complications of Type 2 Diabetes

Remember that when your type 2 diabetes is well managed, your risk of complications is very low. Good blood glucose management is a big part of this process, but there's often quite a bit more involved. People living with type 2 diabetes often must pay extra attention to their blood pressure and cholesterol levels and may require various forms of medication, depending on the severity of the condition.

The human body is very sensitive to blood glucose levels that remain out of the normal range for an extended period of time because these excess sugars can damage bodily organs, including the heart, eyes, kidneys, nerves (such as in your feet), and even your sexual organs.

While you will have to work closely with your health care team to determine the best way to navigate these risks on an individual level, I've gone to great lengths to ensure the dietary guidance to follow takes into consideration as many of these concerns as possible.

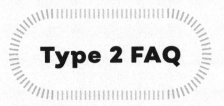

Type 2 FAQ

Does exercise help with type 2 diabetes, and how much should I aim for?

Regular physical activity can work in tandem with a healthy diet to improve blood glucose levels and reduce blood pressure and risk of cardiovascular disease. An ideal to work toward would be around 150 minutes of aerobic exercise per week (e.g., run, jog, walk, bike, swim), broken up into 30-minute sessions (five times a week) and incorporating some resistance training (e.g., using weights, push-ups) and stretching exercises (e.g., yoga).

Do I need to take insulin with type 2 diabetes?

Insulin is not the go-to first-line medication in most circumstances for those who are newly diagnosed with type 2 diabetes. If other management strategies (such as dietary modification) and other medications (such as metformin) do not yield positive results, it is possible for someone living with type 2 to eventually require insulin. This is a decision that is made by you and your medical care team based on a wide variety of personal factors and health-related considerations that go beyond the scope of this book.

What role does stress play in type 2 diabetes?

Mindfulness practices, such as meditation, may have a role to play for those living with type 2 diabetes who are suffering emotional distress. A 2013 study out of the *Diabetes Care* journal found that such practices, while not improving blood glucose control, did improve measures of mental health and quality of life in those living with type 2 diabetes.

A Healthy Diet While Living with Type 2

Alongside the guidance and support of your health care team, a proper understanding of some fundamental nutrition principles will go a long way to improving your quality of life while living with type 2 diabetes.

In my private practice, I often encounter individuals with newly diagnosed type 2 diabetes who believe their first course of action is to completely avoid or minimize carbohydrates. It's important for you to realize right off the bat that this is not a dietary principle that is widely adopted by reputable diabetes management organizations, and many people living with type 2 diabetes achieve good blood sugar control and optimal health while consuming carbohydrates. In fact, many of the most nutrient-dense and heart-healthy foods—including fruits, vegetables, legumes, and whole grains—contain carbs.

That being said, the types and amounts of carbohydrates you eat do matter, since carbohydrate-containing foods play a significant role in dictating your body's blood glucose levels. Understanding carbohydrates is not the same as avoiding them, and to explore this distinction further, we have to start by discussing what is meant by the term *glycemic index*.

Glycemic Index

The glycemic index, also known as GI, is a very important concept for people living with type 2 diabetes to be aware of. The GI of a food is rated on a scale between 0 and 100 and essentially measures how a food affects your blood sugar levels.

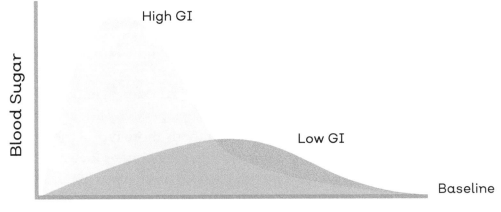

Does a food raise your blood sugar level quickly and sharply? Or does it raise it in a more delayed, sustained fashion? Sharp changes in blood sugar levels that arise from high glycemic index foods are not ideal, especially in the context of someone living with type 2 diabetes.

The GI rating of a food depends on several factors, including the amount of carbohydrate it contains, the amount and type of fiber it contains, the presence of other macronutrients (e.g., fat, protein), and how it is cooked/prepared. Baked goods made from white flour (e.g., white bread, muffins, bagels, etc.), white rice, instant oatmeal, and mashed potatoes are examples of foods that tend to have a high GI rating and the potential to raise blood sugar levels quite sharply.

On the other side of the spectrum, foods like nuts, seeds, legumes, and whole grains like barley, quinoa, and steel-cut oatmeal have a much lower rating. A 2002 *American Journal of Clinical Nutrition* paper firmly stated that replacing high GI foods with lower to moderate GI foods is an important step for improving blood sugar management, and that sentiment is echoed to this day.

Although you don't always have to avoid higher GI foods, Michelle and I have endeavored to incorporate as many lower glycemic index ingredients as possible into the recipes for exactly this reason.

The "Standard" American Diet

One of the big goals of this book is to help you understand that you can still enjoy your favorite foods as someone with type 2 diabetes. Very often the term "standard American diet" is used in a derogatory fashion, but I'm looking at it more from the perspective of how we can make some of the most popular American foods more type 2 friendly.

Polls today indicate that some of the foods Americans love most include pizza, tacos, pasta, and hamburgers. From the lens of blood glucose management, there are a few important connections between all of these foods: They usually include high glycemic index ingredients made from white flour, and they can contain high levels of sodium and saturated fat, which aren't great for cardiovascular health in large quantities. My co-author Michelle and I have you covered, though, as a number of recipes in the pages to come are diabetes- and heart-friendly re-creations of your favorite dishes.

And what about America's favorite vegetable? Did you know that according to USDA data, the humble potato is the most consumed vegetable in the United States? Potatoes are a very interesting topic as they relate to the glycemic index, specifically because a mashed potato served piping hot will have a very high GI, whereas a potato served cold with the skin on (as in a potato salad) has a more moderate GI rating. Squash and sweet potato, which are also in the starchy vegetable family, actually have low GI scores despite the fact that they are sweeter-tasting foods.

Many people automatically assume all things sweet or that contain any sugar at all must be completely avoided if you have diabetes. As you can see from the example above, and as I will demonstrate further in the sections to come, that's not necessarily the case.

Supplements and Type 2 Diabetes

For many people, the supplement industry represents a quick fix or expedited path toward one's health goals. As a dietitian, I can more than appreciate the fact that turning to supplements can be tempting, especially when you first receive a potentially startling medical diagnosis.

The reality is, however, that the state of scientific evidence around supplements and blood sugar management really isn't great. There is one exception, though: psyllium fiber.

Psyllium is a special type of plant fiber often sold in a powdered form at your local health food or grocery store, or you can find it online via Amazon or other outlets. A 2019 study out of the *Diabetes Care* journal found that 1 to 2 tablespoons of psyllium fiber daily can contribute to improvements in fasting blood glucose and A1C scores in individuals living with type 2 diabetes. It's also effective at lowering blood cholesterol levels, which is another important consideration for people living with type 2 diabetes. Psyllium can be consumed mixed with water or added to foods like oatmeal or yogurt. It's also one of the ingredients in Kellogg's All-Bran Buds.

Quick Fixes vs. Long-Term Vision

I next want to touch upon the importance of adopting a mid- to long-term vision when it comes to managing type 2 diabetes as well as your general health while living with type 2. I'm sure that many of you reading this book will have spent at least some time searching online and reading up on diabetes management solutions, not of all which are accurate (unfortunately). Very often these solutions are presented in the forms of expensive supplements or overly restrictive diets.

I won't go so far as to say these types of diets don't work for some people, but let's be honest: They are not sustainable or enjoyable for a large portion of the population, and we always need to keep in mind that good health comes from what you eat, not what you don't.

One of the big markers of blood sugar management in type 2 diabetes is A1C, and it's often measured every three months. While A1C targets are often personalized, the American Diabetes Association generally states that the A1C goal for most adults living with diabetes is less than 7 percent. Optimizing your nutrition has the potential to ultimately reduce your current A1C by between 1 and 2 percentage points, but these changes must be maintained to keep it down—hence why a long-term view to the sustainability of your approach is so important.

Key Foods and Nutrients

Up to this point, I've given you some hints as to my nutrition philosophy when it comes to type 2 diabetes. In this section, we will take things to the next level and really home in on the key foods and nutrients that play the biggest role on your path toward better health.

Keep in mind that for most people living with diabetes, managing blood pressure and cholesterol are also important considerations due to an elevated risk of heart disease. The vast majority of the foods listed in this section, which are very useful for diabetes management, also have the nutritional characteristics to support good blood pressure and blood cholesterol management. That's the beautiful thing about truly nutrient-dense foods—they serve multiple purposes in the human body.

BEANS, PEAS, AND LENTILS

From the culinary perspective, the term *pulse* refers to the family of foods including various types of beans, peas, and lentils such as chickpeas, black beans, kidney beans, and so on. In my professional experience, the pulse family of foods tend to be underestimated, and yet a 2018 paper out of the *Journal of Clinical Nutrition* clearly demonstrated that people who consume more legumes tend to have a lower risk of type 2 diabetes. They are also of great benefit to those living with type 2 diabetes because, of all carbohydrate-containing foods, pulses have the most minimal impact on blood sugar levels, reflecting a low glycemic index and high fiber and protein content.

According to a 2016 *Canadian Journal of Diabetes* study, an average of 5 cups of pulses per week over several weeks can significantly improve blood sugar control in people living with diabetes. The regular inclusion of pulses is a fundamental management strategy for type 2 diabetes, and you will notice that foods from this group are heavily featured throughout the recipe section of the book for this reason. I recommend purchasing low-sodium canned versions whenever possible to keep sodium intake down.

NUTS AND OTHER HEART-HEALTHY FATS

Nuts and seeds are another fundamental group of foods that I consider underrated and generally underappreciated. In fact, they are a fundamentally important food for optimal heart health and good blood sugar management. Their cardiovascular benefits stem from large amounts of blood pressure–lowering minerals (e.g., calcium, magnesium, potassium) as well as their monounsaturated ("healthy") fat content, which helps contribute to lower cholesterol levels.

According to a comprehensive 2014 review out of the *PLoS One* journal, you are looking at consuming around ⅓ cup (50 grams, 1.75 ounces) of nuts daily to make the most of their positive effects on blood glucose levels. For those who can't consume nuts for allergy or preferential reasons, avocado and seeds are great alternatives that are very similar nutritionally. I suggest avoiding salted varieties to help keep sodium intake down.

PLANT PROTEIN

Plant protein is a general categorization of foods of plant origin that have a meaningful amount of protein and iron. Legumes, nuts, and seeds, which I've discussed above, all count in this category, as do soy-based foods such as tofu, tempeh, edamame, and soy milk—in addition to the host of plant-based meat alternative products now widely available.

Why do I bring this up? Well, plant protein sources tend to be very high in fiber, which explains why a 2015 study out of the *Nutrients* journal found that individuals living with diabetes who swapped in more plant proteins tended to have better blood sugar control. If you aren't familiar with cooking using a plant-based protein source, the vegan/vegetarian recipe chapter has you covered (see page 103).

ANIMAL PROTEIN

Animal protein, especially from lean sources like poultry and omega-3 rich sources like salmon and sardines, also play an important role in a balanced diet for most omnivorous people. Milk, yogurt, and red meat also have a part to play, although lower-fat versions are preferable, when possible, to moderate the saturated fat content of the diet.

I should note that dairy and dairy alternatives (such as soy milk) tend to be high in blood pressure–lowering minerals like calcium and potassium. Regardless of the protein type, the inclusion of protein in a meal slows down the rate at which it is digested and leads to a smaller increase in blood sugar levels. That's why most recipes in our book contain at least one source of protein, whether it be of plant or animal origin.

VEGETABLES

It probably won't surprise you to hear me say that a diet rich in vegetables is a cornerstone of good health for just about anyone, including those living with type 2 diabetes.

The regular inclusion of multiple daily servings of vegetables has the potential to improve your A1C as well as reduce your blood pressure and blood cholesterol levels owing to the significant amount of fiber, vitamins, minerals, and antioxidants that they contain.

So how many veggies do you need to get the benefit? A 2012 study published in *Geriatrics and Gerontology International* looking at older adults in Japan found that consuming a minimum of 2½ ounces of green vegetables daily led to significant improvements in A1C levels. That's a great starting point!

FRUIT

Fruit is very misunderstood when it comes to the world of diabetes management. Some people hold the erroneous belief that fruit must be removed from the diet to improve blood sugar control, but a 2013 study published in *Nutrition Journal* found that cutting out fruit did not improve A1C levels. Fruit remains a natural source of sweetness, vitamins, minerals, antioxidants, and fiber that can and should play a meaningful role in blood sugar management. A 2013 study in *Complementary Therapies in Clinical Practice* found that people living with diabetes consuming 17.5 ounces of strawberries daily experienced decreases in A1C over a six-week period.

The sodium content of your diet is a relevant consideration because people living with type 2 diabetes are more likely to have high blood pressure, which can be further increased by excess dietary sodium. Foods that tend to be highest in sodium include those ordered out (e.g., pizza, pasta), frozen meals, and processed meats (e.g., ham, salami, etc.), as well as certain condiments, salad dressings, sauces, and spices.

Cooking more meals at home, like the ones in this book, and choosing low-sodium versions of products will go a long way toward reducing your daily sodium intake.

Meal Times

The importance of meal timing is one of those topics that is often overstated in most contexts, but diabetes management is not one of them.

Being consistent in how you space out your meals throughout the day, and day to day, can help improve your blood sugar control in the long term. What this means for you in your day-to-day life is following a similar eating schedule from one day to the next and eating similar amounts of food, specifically carbohydrates, at each meal. The recipes in the book are optimized for this very purpose.

Hydration

Water and beverage recommendations can vary based on multiple factors, but unless you've been medically advised otherwise, reasonable targets include two liters daily for adult women and three liters daily for adult men, with the rest coming from the naturally occurring water content of your food. These values also include water coming from coffee, tea, and other beverages.

A 2017 study out of the *Nutrition Research* journal found that multiple days in a row of low water intake has the potential to negatively affect blood sugar control, so hydration is certainly something to stay on top of. Sparkling water, water with a touch of lemon, or carbonated beverages that are sugar-free are also reasonable places to look to increase your water intake.

Should You Worry About Added or Hidden Sugars?

I know this is a topic that concerns some of my clients, but the idea of added sugars in foods is actually not something I want you to focus on too much. I'd rather you instead think more about the glycemic index as well as the source and quantity of your carbohydrate intake.

Products like white bread, for example, may not contain much sugar at all but can still raise blood sugar levels much more sharply than, for example, a high-protein flavored Greek yogurt that has both naturally occurring and added sugar. Be aware of added sugars, but I recommend placing the majority of your efforts on understanding food and the glycemic index.

How to Build Your Plate

FRUIT
1 SERVING

MEAT &
ALTERNATIVES

VEGETABLES

RICE &
ALTERNATIVES

The majority of the recipes in this book are based on a fundamental plate-building strategy that emphasizes a ratio of 50 percent veggies, 25 percent starches/carbs, and 25 percent protein.

Veggies: This category refers specifically to non-starchy vegetables such as broccoli, leafy greens, tomatoes, bell peppers, Brussels sprouts, zucchini, bok choy, cauliflower—and the list goes on. These types of foods contain an incredible amount of antioxidants, vitamins, and minerals, and their high-fiber content means they have a strong slowing effect on how quickly the food we eat ends up as sugar in our bloodstream.

Protein: Protein from a variety of sources is an important consideration for a healthy, balanced plate. Different types of protein sources offer their own unique benefits; for example, fish is particularly high in vitamin D and omega-3s. Other protein resources we will rely on in this book include poultry, tofu, eggs, and red meat. Protein has an important role to play in keeping us satiated after a meal, and, like fiber, it helps slow down the speed at which our body processes a meal.

Starches/Carbs: Starchy carbohydrate-containing foods come from multiple food groups, including starchy vegetables (e.g., sweet potato, squash, potato), whole grains (e.g., bread, brown rice, quinoa, barley), and legumes (e.g., lentils, chickpeas, kidney beans). The focal point for good blood sugar management in type 2 diabetes trends toward the higher fiber and lower glycemic index carbs mentioned.

Set Yourself Up for Success

Now that we've gone through some of the nutrition science, it's time to start moving from the theoretical to the practical, where we discuss how you can truly start to utilize my suggestions in your daily life.

The recipes here will play a big role in that process, but before you can truly dive into them, you will need to optimize your food environment for success. This is just a fancy way of saying make sure your kitchen and pantry are stocked with the foods and ingredients you need to thrive.

The staples listed in this section are not only invaluable tools, but also used frequently throughout the recipe section. Notice the emphasis on 100 percent whole-grain products, given the fact that items made from entirely refined flour (such as certain types of bread, crackers, and baked goods) tend to have a high glycemic index. These are foods that we want to swap with whole-grain alternatives when possible.

Pantry

- ▶ All-natural peanut butter or almond butter
- ▶ Almond flour
- ▶ Brown rice
- ▶ Cider or balsamic vinegar
- ▶ Cocoa powder
- ▶ Light coconut milk
- ▶ Low-sodium broth (chicken, vegetable)
- ▶ Low-sodium tamari or soy sauce
- ▶ Nuts (almonds, pecans, cashews, walnuts, pistachios)
- ▶ Oats (rolled, steel cut)
- ▶ Oils (olive, sesame)
- ▶ Olives

- Pulse (lentils, chickpeas, kidney beans, black beans, great northern beans)
- Quinoa
- Seeds (chia, sesame, flaxseed, sunflower, pumpkin)
- Tomatoes (no-salt-added), diced and crushed
- Unsweetened protein powder
- Whole-grain bread, pita, or tortillas
- Whole-grain pasta

Refrigerator/Freezer

- Eggs
- Extra-firm tofu
- Frozen fish
- Frozen fruit (strawberries, avocados, raspberries, peaches, bananas, mangoes)
- Frozen veggies (spinach, kale, cauliflower rice, edamame, peas)
- Low-fat cheese (Cheddar, Parmesan)
- Low-fat plain Greek yogurt
- Low-sodium feta
- Unsweetened non-dairy milk (almond, cashew, oat)

Satisfying Cravings

Craving is a word that gets thrown around a lot. It essentially refers to an intense desire for a specific food or type of food within a group of similar foods. Cravings can occur in a variety of contexts, including hunger, stress, and excessive food restriction.

We've been careful to include modified versions of many people's favorite dishes in this book to help you avoid cravings that may be brought about by restricting what you eat. It's also important to note that many of the meals and ingredients that are blood sugar friendly are also particularly satiating, meaning they will really help manage your hunger levels between meals.

Even so, desires for certain sweet, savory, or salty foods may arise from time to time. Here are some simple, fun snack ideas that all contain a low or moderate amount of GI carbohydrates.

Sweet: 2 cups of frozen berries

Savory: 2 cups of microwave or air-popped popcorn

Sweet and savory: 1 banana with 1 tablespoon peanut butter

Salty: ¾ cup home-roasted chickpeas

Meals in 30 Minutes

If you're anything like me when it comes to time spent in the kitchen, you probably want the most results for the least time and effort possible. That's why 30-minute meals are a foundational theme of the book.

You really don't need your path to healthier eating to involve three times more energy in the kitchen. With that in mind, let's chat about a few time-saving tactics that will really help you flourish in the recipe chapters to come.

Time-Saving Cooking Strategies

Here are a few quick tips to help save you time in the kitchen.

Start Strong: Have all the ingredients you need organized in front of you before starting a recipe to avoid wasting time and energy going back and forth from the refrigerator or pantry.

Choose Wisely: The recipes in this book are all curated to be 30-minute meals, but some may use ingredients or cooking styles that you are more comfortable with—start with those.

Chop, Chop: The more finely you chop ingredients, the quicker they will cook, so if you see an opportunity to take advantage of this, be sure to do so!

Slow Down Your Eating

A recently published 2020 study from the *Nutrients* journal found that a reduction in eating time for a meal from 20 to 10 minutes can lead to higher blood sugar readings after eating.

Many people rush their meals—or, as I say to my clients, try to eat a meal that should take 15 minutes in 5 minutes. If you find yourself in this position more often than not, I urge you to consider slowing down.

Make Use of Appliances

Certain recipes in this book can be prepared more quickly when taking advantage of unique appliances like a slow cooker, blender, Instant Pot, air fryer, or even the microwave.

You won't necessarily need any of the above to prep the meals, but if you do have these appliances around, use them. They will make preparing meals easier.

Another tip I'd like to give you is not to underestimate your freezer. Keeping frozen fruits and vegetables means you always have fresh ingredients on hand.

Take Advantage of Healthy Convenience Foods

There are certain convenience foods and ingredients that you can really utilize to save time and energy throughout the meal-prep process.

These include:

- ▶ Boxed, prewashed leafy greens (spinach, spring mix)
- ▶ Cubed squash or sweet potatoes
- ▶ Greek yogurt
- ▶ Sliced bell peppers
- ▶ Sliced mushrooms
- ▶ Microwaveable veggie bags
- ▶ Minced garlic and ginger
- ▶ Roasted chickpea or lentil snacks
- ▶ Seasoned sunflower seeds
- ▶ Store-bought no-sodium seasoning blends

Make-Ahead

For many people, including a significant number of my clients, having a game plan for the week ahead is often the crucial factor that allows them to eat in the way they intend.

There are a few things that will help put you in a position of success from this perspective:

Make Grocery Trips Count: As you adapt to a new style of cooking that is heavily based on having certain ingredients, it will be increasingly important for you to have a very good idea of what you plan to cook the week ahead and thus know which ingredients you will need to buy to make that happen.

Look Out for "Make-Ahead" Recipes: Several recipes in this book come equipped with Make-Ahead tips, which will teach you some culinary tricks to prep parts of the recipe in advance and save you some cooking time down the line.

Don't Forget the Balanced-Plate Model: Remember that if life gets in the way on any given day, which happens to the best of us, you can always default to the balanced-plate model as a meal-planning guide. If you keep the staple and convenience foods around that I've suggested, you will always be able to prepare a balanced meal if you really want to.

About the Recipes

If I've done my job thus far, you've arrived at the end of this chapter with the knowledge and confidence that eating in a way to optimize your health and blood sugar levels is firmly within your grasp.

Michelle has written the delicious recipes that follow, but rest assured that she and I have worked very closely to ensure that the recipes in this book will allow you to leverage all the nutrition science I've discussed so far. Our aim is also to allow you to do so in a time-friendly and practical way.

Recipe Labels

To accommodate the health- and/or preference-driven dietary restrictions of a wide range of readers, certain recipes in the book have special labels to help you quickly identify characteristics of the dish.

Dairy-Free: Recipes are free from milk, cheese, yogurt, and other related products but may include eggs.

Gluten-Free: Recipes are free from gluten-containing ingredients such as wheat and related products. Always check ingredient packaging for gluten-free labeling to ensure that foots, especially oats, were processed in a completely gluten-free facility.

Vegetarian: Recipes do not include any red meat, fish, or poultry but may include eggs and/or dairy.

Vegan: Recipes do not include any products of animal origin and exclude eggs and dairy.

Carb Content

Up until this point, I've focused primarily on the type of foods, and particularly carbohydrate-containing foods, that are most helpful to optimize blood sugar control and overall health. This is a very relevant consideration for people living with type 2 diabetes, but so, too, is the amount of carbohydrate that you consume at each meal. In fact, this is a very important consideration and one that I know is probably on your mind.

As I've mentioned, it's best to consume carbohydrates in consistent amounts across your daily meals, and in consistent amounts from day to day as well. The extent to which your carbohydrate intake needs to be monitored will depend on several variables, including the guidance of your health care team, the severity of your diabetes, and the amount/type of medication you may be on. On top of individual variation in caloric needs, the right number of carbohydrates per day and per meal can look very different for different people.

To establish a reasonable baseline, what we've used the FDA general guideline of 2,000 calories per day and assumed a reasonable calorie contribution from carbohydrates to be 50 percent of daily caloric intake. This gives us a total of 250 grams of carbohydrate per day to work with, which is an average of 75 grams of carbohydrate per meal (assuming someone eats three meals per day), leaving about 25 grams for a single daily snack.

Using this math, we've endeavored to set all recipes that could serve as meals to 75 grams of net carbohydrate, which is equal to the total carbohydrate content of the recipe minus the fiber content. We exclude fiber from this calculation because it does not contribute to raising blood sugar levels.

Tips

As a final little note before you get to the good stuff, some recipes you encounter will also have special tips that fall into one of three categories.

Keep your eyes peeled as these tips will help make the food preparation experience that much better.

Make-Ahead: These time-saving tips will teach you how to make a portion or all of the recipe ahead of time for storage/freezing before cooking.

Variation: These tips will offer substitution suggestions to either allow a dish to better meet your dietary preferences, or just to spice it up from the original version.

Prep Tip: These tips will offer little tricks or strategies to make the cooking process quicker and easier.

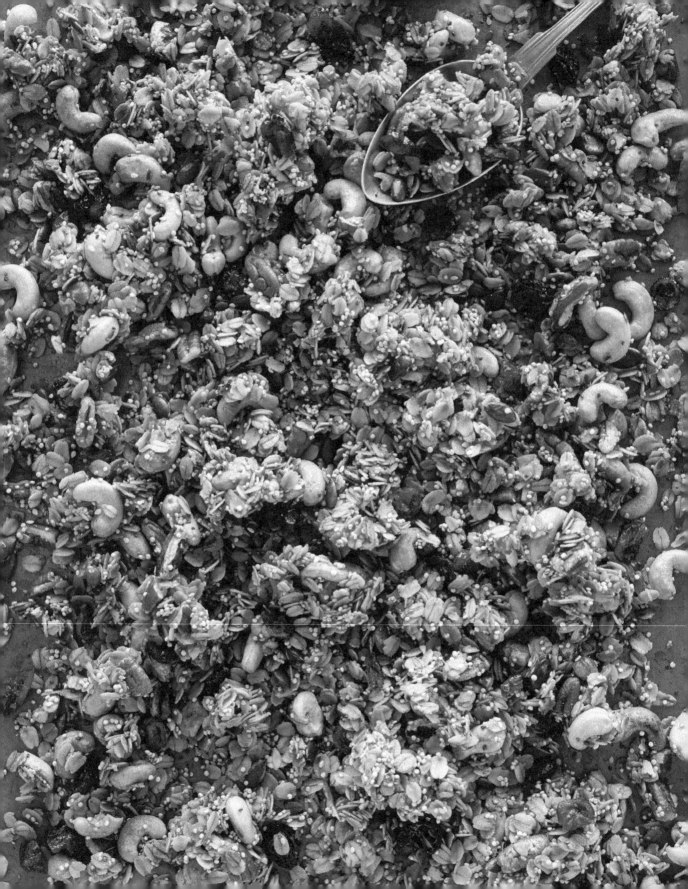

BREAKFAST AND BRUNCH

Spinach-Avocado Smoothie

GLUTEN-FREE, VEGAN **PREP TIME:** 5 minutes **SERVES** 2

Adding avocado to this berry-and-green-packed smoothie creates a luscious milkshake-like texture that lasts overnight in the refrigerator. The healthy fat and fiber in this fruit can help prevent spikes in blood sugar. If you prefer, you can omit the protein powder and use a half cup of low-fat Greek yogurt for a tart-sweet taste.

2 cups unsweetened non-dairy milk

2 cups baby spinach

1 cup frozen strawberries

½ avocado, peeled and pitted

2 scoops unsweetened vegan protein powder

2 teaspoons pure vanilla extract

Place the milk, spinach, strawberries, avocado, protein powder, and vanilla in a blender and blend until smooth. Serve.

MAKE-AHEAD: *You can store this smoothie in the refrigerator overnight in a sealed container. Just stir or shake before serving.*

Per Serving: Calories: 309; Total fat: 11g; Saturated fat: 2g; Sodium: 198mg; Carbohydrates: 25g; Sugar: 6g; Fiber: 7g; Protein: 26g

Raspberry-Ricotta Smoothie

GLUTEN-FREE, VEGETARIAN **PREP TIME:** 5 minutes **SERVES** 2

Cheese in a smoothie? Yes indeed! Mild ricotta combined with raspberries, banana, and kale creates a filling, protein-packed smoothie that might become your new favorite. Raspberries are low on the glycemic index and high in fiber. If you don't have frozen berries, substitute fresh and add a couple ice cubes.

2 cups unsweetened non-dairy milk

1 cup low-fat ricotta cheese

1 cup frozen raspberries

1 cup chopped baby kale

½ banana

1 teaspoon pure vanilla extract

Pinch ground cinnamon

Place the milk, ricotta, raspberries, kale, banana, vanilla, and cinnamon in a blender and blend until smooth. Serve immediately.

Per Serving: Calories: 324; Total fat: 14g; Saturated fat: 6g; Sodium: 202mg; Carbohydrates: 26g; Sugar: 8g; Fiber: 7g; Protein: 23g

Spiced Seeds and Nuts Granola

GLUTEN-FREE, VEGAN **PREP TIME:** 5 minutes **COOK TIME:** 25 minutes **SERVES** 8

Homemade granola is a versatile, low-sugar addition to yogurt, smoothie bowls, or as a stand-alone meal topped with a splash of your favorite milk. The cinnamon in this recipe adds flavor, and can also help decrease fasting sugar levels.

2 cups gluten-free rolled oats

½ cup raw sunflower seeds

½ cup shredded unsweetened coconut

½ cup chopped pecans

½ cup slivered almonds

¼ cup maple syrup

2 tablespoons canola oil

½ teaspoon ground cinnamon

¼ teaspoon ground nutmeg

⅛ teaspoon sea salt

1. Preheat the oven to 300°F and line a baking sheet with parchment paper. Set it aside.

2. In a large bowl, toss together the oats, sunflower seeds, coconut, pecans, and almonds until mixed.

3. In a small bowl, whisk the maple syrup, oil, cinnamon, nutmeg, and salt until blended.

4. Add the maple syrup mixture to the oat mixture and mix until very well coated.

5. Spread the oat mixture on the baking sheet and bake for about 25 minutes, stirring frequently, until the granola is golden brown and crunchy.

6. Let the granola cool, break up the large pieces, and store in an airtight container in the refrigerator or freezer for up to 1 month.

Per Serving: Calories: 289; Total fat: 18g; Saturated fat: 3g; Sodium: 43mg; Carbohydrates: 25g; Sugar: 7g; Fiber: 5g; Protein: 7g

Lemon-Blueberry Overnight Oats

GLUTEN-FREE, VEGETARIAN **PREP TIME:** 5 minutes, plus sitting overnight
SERVES 2

I remember when I discovered overnight oats. I was on a trip to Germany, and my lovely hostess at a charming bed and breakfast served a creamy fruit-and-seed topped cold oatmeal every morning. I've added chia seeds to this version because they contain heaps of fiber that can control blood glucose levels and keep you full for hours.

½ cup milk of choice

½ cup low-fat plain Greek yogurt

½ cup gluten-free rolled oats

2 tablespoons chia seeds

Juice and zest of 1 lemon

1 tablespoon maple syrup

1 teaspoon pure vanilla extract

Pinch sea salt

1 cup blueberries

1. In a medium bowl, whisk the milk, yogurt, oats, chia seeds, lemon juice, lemon zest, maple syrup, vanilla, and salt.

2. Fold in the blueberries, cover, and refrigerate for at least 4 hours or overnight.

MAKE-AHEAD: *Double the recipe, evenly divide the ingredients among four jars, seal, and refrigerate for a convenient grab-and-go breakfast.*

Per Serving: Calories: 283; Total fat: 6g; Saturated fat: 1g; Sodium: 133mg; Carbohydrates: 42g; Sugar: 17g; Fiber: 10g; Protein: 10g

Strawberry and Ricotta Pancakes

VEGETARIAN PREP TIME: 10 minutes **COOK TIME:** 20 minutes **SERVES** 4

*Pancakes seem to be a lazy weekend morning meal—
decadent and time-consuming—but they don't need to be.
This healthy, speedy version features fresh strawberries,
tangy ricotta, whole-wheat flour, and a hint of lemon and
vanilla to tie the flavors together. Double the recipe and try
these cold with a bit of almond butter for a tempting snack.*

**1¼ cups milk
of choice**

**½ cup low-fat
ricotta cheese**

1 large egg

**1 tablespoon
canola oil**

**1 tablespoon freshly
squeezed lemon juice**

**½ teaspoon pure
vanilla extract**

**1¼ cups
whole-wheat flour**

1 tablespoon sugar

1. In a large bowl, whisk the milk, ricotta, egg, oil, lemon juice, and vanilla until well blended.

2. Whisk in the flour, sugar, baking powder, and salt until combined.

3. Heat a griddle or large skillet on medium heat and lightly grease it with oil. Reduce the heat to medium-low and, working in batches, add the batter in ¼-cup measures.

4. Cook until the edges of the pancakes are firm and golden, about 2 minutes, then scatter the strawberries on top of each, and flip.

**2 teaspoons
baking powder**

¼ teaspoon salt

**Canola oil,
for cooking**

**1 cup sliced
strawberries**

5. Cook the pancakes for 1 minute more until cooked through, transfer them to a plate, and cover loosely with aluminum foil to keep them warm. Repeat with the remaining batter and serve.

VARIATION: *Instead of cooking the strawberries into the pancakes, you can use the fruit for a topping instead. Any fruit—such as peaches, blueberries, or raspberries—would be delicious.*

Per Serving: Calories: 285; Total fat: 9g; Saturated fat: 2g; Sodium: 220mg; Carbohydrates: 40g; Sugar: 9g; Fiber: 5g; Protein: 12g

Shakshuka

DAIRY-FREE, GLUTEN-FREE, VEGETARIAN **PREP TIME:** 10 minutes
COOK TIME: 20 minutes **SERVES** 4

I spent several years working as a chef in North Africa, and this delicious dish always had top billing on my restaurant menu. The spicy veggie tomato sauce is the perfect vehicle to poach eggs. Add a chopped jalapeño pepper to boost the heat. Serve with a slice of whole-grain toast or pita bread for a satisfying meal.

2 tablespoons olive oil

1 red bell pepper, seeded and chopped

1 onion, diced

1 tablespoon minced garlic

1 (28-ounce) can no-salt-added diced tomatoes, drained

1 teaspoon paprika

1 teaspoon ground cumin

½ teaspoon chili powder

8 large eggs

¼ cup chopped fresh parsley, for garnish

1. In a large skillet, heat the oil over medium-high heat.

2. Sauté the bell pepper, onion, and garlic for about 4 minutes, until softened.

3. Stir in the tomatoes, paprika, cumin, and chili powder and simmer for 10 minutes.

4. Use the back of a spoon to make 8 wells, then crack an egg into each well. Cover the skillet and let the eggs cook for about 6 minutes, until the whites are no longer translucent.

5. Serve topped with parsley.

MAKE-AHEAD: *Make the sauce ahead and reheat over medium heat in a skillet. Continue the recipe at step 4*

Per Serving: Calories: 263; Total fat: 17g; Saturated fat: 4g; Sodium: 178mg; Carbohydrates: 14g; Sugar: 8g; Fiber: 5g; Protein: 15g

Apple and Cheddar Omelet

GLUTEN-FREE, VEGETARIAN **PREP TIME:** 10 minutes **COOK TIME:** 10 minutes
SERVES 2

Apple and Cheddar is a classic pairing because the sweet fruit and slightly salty cheese complement one another. Combining them in a fluffy omelet with kale and thyme creates a unique, delicious dish ideal for guests or a leisurely weekend meal. Other cheeses such as Gruyère, Swiss, or Havarti work as well.

Nonstick
cooking spray

4 large eggs

**2 tablespoons milk
of choice**

**¼ teaspoon chopped
fresh thyme**

Sea salt

**Freshly ground
black pepper**

**1 apple, cored
and chopped**

½ cup chopped kale

**¼ cup shredded
low-fat
Cheddar cheese**

1. Spray a medium skillet with cooking spray and place it on medium-high heat.

2. In a small bowl, whisk the eggs, milk, and thyme and season with salt and pepper.

3. Pour the egg mixture into the skillet, swirling it gently to move the eggs around. Cook until the eggs are mostly set, and then sprinkle the apple, kale, and Cheddar evenly over the surface.

4. When the eggs are cooked through and the Cheddar is melted, fold one side over the other, cut it in half, and serve.

Per Serving: Calories: 259; Total fat: 13g; Saturated fat: 4g; Sodium: 243mg; Carbohydrates: 15g; Sugar: 11g; Fiber: 2g; Protein: 17g

Breakfast Bruschetta

VEGETARIAN **PREP TIME:** 10 minutes **COOK TIME:** 15 minutes **SERVES** 4

Bruschetta is a traditional Italian appetizer made of grilled bread topped with tomatoes, onions, herbs, and garlic. This breakfast version uses English muffins instead, and scrambled eggs are added to the savory tomato mixture. You can make the topping ahead and store it until you are serving the meal.

2 large tomatoes, chopped

¼ red onion, finely chopped

2 tablespoons finely chopped fresh basil

2 tablespoons olive oil

½ teaspoon minced garlic

Sea salt

Freshly ground black pepper

4 whole-wheat English muffins, split

1. Preheat the oven to 400°F. Line a small baking sheet with parchment paper.

2. In a small bowl, mix the tomatoes, red onion, basil, oil, and garlic. Season with salt and pepper.

3. Place the English muffins on the baking sheet and evenly top the halves with the bruschetta mixture. Bake for about 10 minutes, until heated through and toasted.

4. While the bruschetta is cooking, in a small bowl, whisk the eggs and season them lightly with salt and pepper.

5. Lightly spray a medium skillet with cooking spray and place it on medium-high heat.

6 large eggs

Nonstick cooking spray

¼ cup shredded Parmesan cheese

6. Pour in the eggs and scramble them for about 2 minutes, until fluffy curds form.

7. Top the English muffins with the eggs, sprinkle with Parmesan cheese, and serve.

VARIATION: *Try adding chopped peaches or nectarines to the bruschetta mixture for a delicious, slightly sweet breakfast.*

Per Serving: Calories: 347; Total fat: 17g; Saturated fat: 4g; Sodium: 487mg; Carbohydrates: 32g; Sugar: 8g; Fiber: 6g; Protein: 18g

Egg and Veggie Quesadillas

VEGETARIAN **PREP TIME:** 10 minutes **COOK TIME:** 15 minutes **SERVES** 2

Quesadillas are often considered a lunch or dinner choice, but they are just as delightful as breakfast. These are inspired by crispy huevos rancheros but you can eat them with your hands like a slice of pizza. The added beans are heart healthy and bring protein and soluble fiber. Try any of your favorite toppings in place of the ones in this recipe. I like sliced pickled jalapeño, fresh tomatoes, and a generous splash of hot sauce.

Nonstick cooking spray

4 large eggs

Sea salt

Freshly ground black pepper

1 teaspoon olive oil

1 red bell pepper, seeded and chopped

1 scallion, both white and green parts, chopped

2 (6-inch) whole-wheat tortillas

½ cup low-sodium canned white beans, drained and rinsed

1. Preheat the oven to 400°F. Grease a large baking sheet with cooking spray.

2. In a small bowl, beat the eggs and season with salt and pepper.

3. In a medium skillet, heat the oil over medium-high heat. Sauté the bell pepper and scallion for about 2 minutes, until softened. Pour in the eggs and scramble for about 3 minutes, until they are fluffy curds.

4. Place the tortillas on the baking sheet and evenly divide the eggs between them, placing them on one-half of each. Top the eggs with the beans, salsa (if using), and Cheddar, and fold the other side of the tortilla over the filling.

¼ cup homemade or
store-bought salsa
(optional)

¼ cup shredded
low-fat
Cheddar cheese

5. Lightly spray the top of the tortilla with cooking spray and bake for about 10 minutes, until the cheese melts and the tortillas are lightly browned. Serve.

Per Serving: Calories: 419; Total fat: 18g; Saturated fat: 6g; Sodium: 567mg; Carbohydrates: 33g; Sugar: 5g; Fiber: 8g; Protein: 23g

Simple Tofu Scramble

GLUTEN-FREE, VEGAN **PREP TIME:** 5 minutes, plus 30 minutes for draining the tofu **COOK TIME:** 10 minutes **SERVES** 2

Many people don't like tofu because it looks intimidating to cook, and if you don't add seasonings, sauces, or marinades, the flavor can be a little flat. Tofu is a spectacular source of protein, though, and the texture is very similar to eggs. The addition of veggies, garlic, and flavor-packed nutritional yeast elevates the recipe to irresistible. To drain the tofu, wrap it in a clean kitchen towel and place it on a plate. Place a heavy can on top and let stand for 30 minutes.

1 (14-ounce) block extra-firm tofu, drained

2 teaspoons olive oil

½ onion, chopped

½ red bell pepper, seeded and chopped

1 teaspoon minced garlic

2 tablespoons nutritional yeast

¼ teaspoon ground turmeric (optional)

Freshly ground black pepper

1. Crumble the drained tofu into a small bowl.

2. In a large skillet, heat the oil over medium-high heat and sauté the onion, bell pepper, and garlic for about 3 minutes, until softened.

3. Add the tofu and sauté for about 4 minutes, until heated through. Stir in the nutritional yeast and turmeric (if using) and toss until the tofu is well coated.

4. Season with pepper and serve.

Per Serving: Calories: 243; Total fat: 16g; Saturated fat: 43g; Sodium: 18mg; Carbohydrates: 9g; Sugar: 3g; Fiber: 2g; Protein: 20g

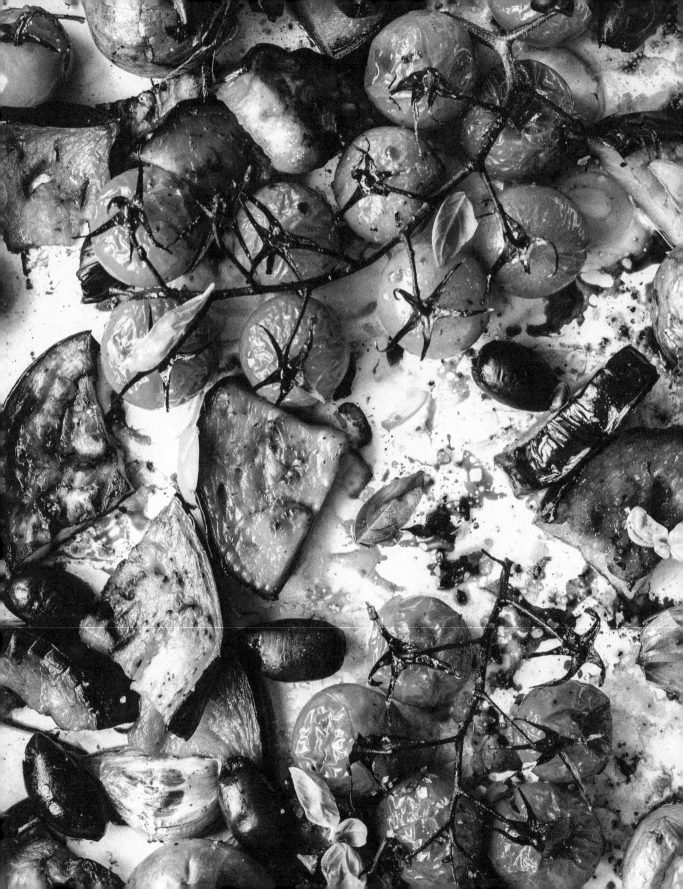

SALADS AND SIDES

Chopped Vegetable-Barley Salad

VEGAN **PREP TIME:** 25 minutes (while the barley cooks) **COOK TIME:** 25 minutes
SERVES 4

This dish has an assortment of wonderful textures from the grains, veggies, and magnesium-rich pumpkin seeds. Magnesium can help regulate blood sugar levels. The beauty of this preparation is that you can complete the rest of the dish while the barley is on the stove. The dressing is just a simple oil and citrus juice blend, but you can use your favorite homemade or store-bought vinaigrette. Just be sure to choose one that is low in added sugar.

1 cup water

½ cup pearl barley

4 cups chopped Brussels sprouts

3 celery stalks, chopped

2 carrots, chopped

1 yellow bell pepper, seeded and chopped chopped

2 cups chopped cauliflower

1 cup halved cherry tomatoes

¼ cup roasted, unsalted pumpkin seeds

1. In a small saucepan, combine the water and barley and bring to a boil over medium-high heat. Cover, reduce the heat to low, and simmer for 22 to 25 minutes, until tender but with a bit of bite.

2. While the barley is cooking, in a large bowl, toss together the Brussels sprouts, celery, carrots, bell pepper, cauliflower, tomatoes, pumpkin seeds, and scallion until well mixed.

3. In a small bowl, whisk the oil and lemon juice and season with salt and pepper.

1 scallion, both white and green parts, chopped

¼ cup extra-virgin olive oil

Juice of 1 lemon

Sea salt

Freshly ground black pepper

4. Add the cooked barley and dressing to the salad, toss to combine, and serve.

PREP TIP: *If you have a food processor, chop all the veggies in it quickly for this tasty dish. The barley can be made ahead and refrigerated for up to 4 days to save even more time.*

Per Serving: Calories: 339; Total fat: 18g; Saturated fat: 3g; Sodium: 115mg; Carbohydrates: 40g; Sugar: 5g; Fiber: 11g; Protein: 10g

Kale Cobb Salad

GLUTEN-FREE **PREP TIME:** 25 minutes **SERVES** 2

Cobb salad is packed with heaps of ingredients, including lettuce, veggies, fruit, poultry, eggs, and cheese. This salad is truly a complete meal! Kale takes the place of chopped romaine to add a boost of protein and iron. This dish is an excellent choice for meal prep—just separate the different components in their own containers or compartments, and then mix before serving.

6 cups torn baby kale, thoroughly washed and dried

½ cup store-bought balsamic dressing or Everyday Balsamic Vinaigrette (page 126)

3 celery stalks, sliced

1 cup chopped cooked store-bought rotisserie chicken

2 hard-boiled eggs, chopped

1 apple, cored and chopped

¼ red onion, chopped

¼ cup crumbled low-fat blue cheese

¼ cup chopped pecans

1. In a large bowl, toss together the kale and dressing. Let stand for 10 minutes.

2. Evenly divide the kale among 4 plates. Top each salad with equal amounts of celery, chicken, eggs, apple, onion, blue cheese, and pecans. Serve immediately.

Per Serving: Calories: 373; Total fat: 16g; Saturated fat: 6g; Sodium: 532mg; Carbohydrates: 34g; Sugar: 16g; Fiber: 6g; Protein: 32g

Autumn-Inspired Fall Slaw

GLUTEN-FREE, VEGAN **PREP TIME:** 30 minutes **SERVES** 4

If you have never eaten raw winter squash before, this salad could be a revelation. The squash is nutrient packed, slightly sweet, and adds a gorgeous color. If you live in an area with pie pumpkins, substitute one for the squash for similar results, and roast the seeds for a tasty topping.

For the dressing

¼ cup extra-virgin olive oil

3 tablespoons apple cider vinegar

1 tablespoon maple syrup

1 teaspoon peeled and grated fresh ginger

For the salad

½ small butternut squash, shredded

¼ head red cabbage, shredded

2 carrots, shredded

1 apple, cored and shredded

2 scallions, both white and green parts, thinly sliced

1 tablespoon chopped fresh thyme

To make the dressing

1. In a small bowl, whisk together the oil, vinegar, maple syrup, and ginger until well blended. Set aside.

To make the salad

2. In a large bowl, toss the squash, red cabbage, carrots, apple, scallions, and thyme until well mixed. Add the dressing, toss, and serve.

VARIATION: *Any type of vegetable will work in this delicious slaw, and you can save time using a pre-shredded store-bought product.*

Per Serving: Calories: 252; Total fat: 17g; Saturated fat: 2g; Sodium: 130mg; Carbohydrates: 24g; Sugar: 17g; Fiber: 4g; Protein: 2g

Spiced Chicken Chickpea Bowls

DAIRY-FREE, GLUTEN-FREE **PREP TIME:** 18 minutes **COOK TIME:** 12 minutes
SERVES 4

A bowl meal is a way to combine flavorful ingredients in one big container; my mother used to call it a "kitchen sink salad" in the '80s (which doesn't trip off the tongue as well). This recipe has a California vibe with avocado, tomatoes, bell pepper, cilantro, and sunflower seeds, and it is packed with filling protein. Don't add the seeds until you are ready to eat, or they will lose their lovely crunch.

1 pound boneless, skinless chicken breast, diced into 1-inch cubes

1 teaspoon ground cumin

Sea salt

Freshly ground black pepper

1 tablespoon olive oil

2 cups canned chickpeas, drained and rinsed

1 English cucumber, cut into ½-inch chunks

1. In a small bowl, toss the chicken chunks with the cumin and season with salt and pepper.

2. In a medium skillet, heat the oil over medium-high heat. Sauté the chicken for about 12 minutes, until it is lightly browned and cooked through.

3. While the chicken is cooking, arrange the chickpeas, cucumber, bell pepper, avocado, and tomatoes in four bowls. Drizzle with the dressing.

1 yellow bell pepper, seeded and cut into ½-inch chunks

1 avocado, peeled, pitted, and chopped

1 cup halved cherry tomatoes

½ cup store-bought balsamic dressing or Everyday Balsamic Vinaigrette (page 126)

¼ cup sunflower seeds

2 tablespoons chopped fresh cilantro

4. Top the bowls with the cooked chicken, sunflower seeds, and cilantro and serve.

VARIATION: *If you want a vegetarian version, omit the chicken and add a cooked grain instead, such as brown rice, farro, or quinoa.*

Per Serving: Calories: 472; Total fat: 20g; Saturated fat: 3g; Sodium: 479mg; Carbohydrates: 41g; Sugar: 8g; Fiber: 12g; Protein: 36g

Lime-Yogurt Cucumber Salad

GLUTEN-FREE, VEGETARIAN **PREP TIME:** 15 minutes, plus 15 minutes draining time
SERVES 4

Sometimes the simplest collection of ingredients creates culinary magic. Who would imagine the humble, low-carb cucumber could sing when mixed with protein-packed yogurt, zesty lime, and fresh mint? The trick to a fabulous cucumber salad is to squeeze out as much liquid as possible, so it doesn't dilute the other flavors or take on a watery consistency.

3 English cucumbers, very thinly sliced

½ teaspoon sea salt

¼ red onion, thinly sliced

½ cup fat-free plain Greek yogurt

2 tablespoons chopped fresh mint, or 1 tablespoon dried mint

Juice and zest of 1 lime

1 tablespoon maple syrup

Freshly ground black pepper

1. Place the cucumber slices in a fine-mesh sieve and toss with the salt. Let the slices sit for 15 minutes to drain out the excess moisture.

2. Transfer the slices to a medium bowl and toss with the onion.

3. In a small bowl, whisk together the yogurt, mint, lime juice, lime zest, and maple syrup.

4. Add the dressing to the cucumber and toss to coat. Season with pepper and serve.

MAKE-AHEAD: *This salad is even better when it sits overnight, so make it the day before to get the best flavor.*

Per Serving: Calories: 62; Total fat: 0g; Saturated fat: 0g; Sodium: 94mg; Carbohydrates: 11g; Sugar: 7g; Fiber: 2g; Protein: 4g

Tabbouleh with Sundried Tomatoes

VEGAN **PREP TIME:** 15 minutes **COOK TIME:** 12 minutes **SERVES** 4

Tabbouleh is a weekly staple in my house, although I sometimes use whole-wheat couscous instead of bulgur. This recipe is very traditional except for the sundried tomatoes, which add a boost of concentrated flavor. I find the intense pop of tomato adds an extra layer to this already flavorful salad.

1½ cups water

¾ cup bulgur

¾ cup chopped marinated sundried tomatoes

1 English cucumber, chopped

¼ red onion, chopped

Juice and zest of 1 lemon

¼ cup chopped fresh parsley

2 tablespoons extra-virgin olive oil

2 tablespoons chopped fresh mint

Sea salt

Freshly ground black pepper

1. In a medium saucepan, bring the water to a boil over high heat. Add the bulgur, cover, reduce the heat to low, and simmer for about 12 minutes, until tender and the water is absorbed. Remove the saucepan from the heat and let stand for 5 minutes, covered.

2. While the bulgur is cooking, in a large bowl, toss the tomatoes, cucumber, onion, lemon juice, lemon zest, parsley, oil, and mint until well mixed.

3. Add the bulgur to the bowl and toss. Season with salt and pepper and serve warm or chilled.

Per Serving: Calories: 194; Total fat: 7g; Saturated fat: 1g; Sodium: 112mg; Carbohydrates: 30g; Sugar: 6g; Fiber: 5g; Protein: 5g

Pesto Zucchini and Carrot "Noodles"

GLUTEN-FREE, VEGAN **PREP TIME:** 15 minutes **COOK TIME:** 2 minutes **SERVES** 4

Don't let the short ingredient list fool you; this is a spectacular-looking and tasting dish. The gorgeous low-calorie vegetable "noodles" are lightly blanched, so they retain their shape, but you can eat them raw to save time. Store-bought pesto is delicious, but you can also use a favorite homemade sauce if you have it stashed in your refrigerator.

4 zucchini, cut into ribbons with a peeler

2 carrots, cut into ribbons with a peeler

¼ cup store-bought vegan basil pesto

1 scallion, both white and green parts, chopped

¼ cup pine nuts

1. Place a large saucepan filled with water on high heat and bring to a boil. Reduce the heat to medium, so the water is simmering, add the zucchini and carrot noodles, and cook for about 2 minutes, until tender-crisp.

2. Drain and transfer the noodles to a serving bowl. Add the pesto and scallion and toss to coat.

3. Top with pine nuts and serve.

PREP TIP: *You can use spiralized vegetables, either homemade or store-bought, instead of making broader "noodles." If using the spiralized veggies, cut the cooking time to about 30 seconds.*

Per Serving: Calories: 189; Total fat: 15g; Saturated fat: 2g; Sodium: 181mg; Carbohydrates: 11g; Sugar: 7g; Fiber: 4g; Protein: 5g

Roasted Brussels Sprouts
with Pumpkin Seeds

GLUTEN-FREE, VEGAN **PREP TIME:** 10 minutes **COOK TIME:** 20 minutes **SERVES** 4

When I was a child, I thought Brussels sprouts were baby cabbages, and I used to eat them by peeling off each tender leaf until the pretty pale-green center remained. I now know that they are a member of the cabbage family, so I was not too far off. Brussels sprouts are an excellent source of vitamins and minerals, including vitamins A, C, and K, iron, and calcium. Take care not to overcook your sprouts—they should be served tender with a bit of bite for best results.

1 pound Brussels sprouts, trimmed and halved lengthwise

1 tablespoon olive oil

Juice and zest of 1 lemon, divided

Sea salt

Freshly ground black pepper

¼ cup roasted, unsalted pumpkin seeds

1. Preheat the oven to 400°F and line a baking sheet with parchment paper.

2. In a large bowl, toss the Brussels sprouts with the oil and lemon juice and season with salt and pepper until well coated.

3. Spread the Brussels sprouts on the baking sheet and bake for 15 to 20 minutes, until lightly caramelized.

4. Toss the Brussels sprouts with the lemon zest and pumpkin seeds and serve.

Per Serving: Calories: 124; Total fat: 7g; Saturated fat: 1g; Sodium: 69mg; Carbohydrates: 12g; Sugar: 3g; Fiber: 5g; Protein: 6g

Quinoa with Chopped Pistachios

GLUTEN-FREE, VEGAN **PREP TIME:** 10 minutes **COOK TIME:** 20 minutes **SERVES** 4

Quinoa is my go-to grain because it cooks quickly and has a wonderful nutty flavor that combines well with everything. Quinoa is high in protein and fiber, which can keep you full for hours. This flavorful recipe makes a perfect side dish for Roasted Spice-Rubbed Pork Tenderloin (page 70) and Sheet-Pan Chicken Parmesan with Cauliflower (page 84). You can also enjoy it alone as a light lunch or dinner.

1 tablespoon olive oil

1 onion, chopped

1 tablespoon minced garlic

1 teaspoon peeled and grated fresh ginger

2 cups low-sodium vegetable broth

1 cup quinoa, rinsed

Sea salt

Freshly ground black pepper

¼ cup chopped roasted pistachios

2 tablespoons chopped fresh parsley

1. In a large saucepan, heat the oil over medium-high heat and sauté the onion, garlic, and ginger for about 3 minutes, until softened.

2. Add the broth and quinoa and bring to a boil. Reduce the heat to low, cover, and simmer for 15 to 17 minutes, or until the liquid is absorbed and the quinoa is tender.

3. Season with salt and pepper and serve topped with pistachios and parsley.

Per Serving: Calories: 245; Total fat: 10g; Saturated fat: 1g; Sodium: 44mg; Carbohydrates: 32g; Sugar: 2g; Fiber: 5g; Protein: 8g

Cauliflower Fried Rice

DAIRY-FREE, GLUTEN-FREE, VEGETARIAN **PREP TIME:** 12 minutes
COOK TIME: 18 minutes **SERVES** 4

Cauliflower rice often finds its way to my table, so I always have frozen packages stacked in the freezer. Using cauliflower instead of rice allows you to enjoy this classic dish without adding too many carbs. This veggie-based dish infused with Asian-inspired flavors is a winner. To make it a complete meal, add chopped cooked chicken or shrimp instead of eggs.

1 tablespoon sesame oil

1 tablespoon minced garlic

2 teaspoons peeled and grated fresh ginger

8 cups riced cauliflower (fresh or frozen)

1 large carrot, shredded

2 cups frozen peas, thawed

2 tablespoons low-sodium soy sauce

2 large eggs, beaten

1 scallion, both white and green parts, thinly sliced

2 teaspoons sesame seeds

1. In a large skillet, heat the oil over medium-high heat. Sauté the garlic and ginger for about 2 minutes, until fragrant.

2. Add the cauliflower and carrot and cook for about 10 minutes, tossing until heated through and the purged liquid evaporates.

3. Add the peas and soy sauce and toss for about 4 minutes, or until mixed and the peas are warmed through.

4. Push the cauliflower rice to the side of the skillet and pour in the eggs. Scramble the eggs for about 2 minutes, and mix them into the rice.

5. Serve topped with scallions and sesame seeds.

Per Serving: Calories: 203; Total fat: 8g; Saturated fat: 2g; Sodium: 373mg; Carbohydrates: 25g; Sugar: 9g; Fiber: 9g; Protein: 12g

Maple Roasted Spaghetti Squash

GLUTEN-FREE, VEGAN **PREP TIME:** 5 minutes **COOK TIME:** 25 minutes **SERVES** 4

Every time I make spaghetti squash, I smile when the pretty strands separate with the fork like bright spaghetti. It is so fun! If you want to enjoy this dish more quickly, place the pierced halves in a microwave-safe dish with a half cup of water and microwave on high for 10 minutes rather than baking in the oven.

1 spaghetti squash, halved lengthwise, seeds and fibers removed

1 teaspoon olive oil

2 tablespoons maple syrup

¼ teaspoon ground nutmeg

¼ teaspoon ground ginger

Sea salt

1. Preheat the oven to 400°F. Line a baking sheet with parchment paper.

2. Rub the cut sides of the squash with the oil and place them hollow-side down on the baking sheet. Pierce the squash several times with a fork.

3. Bake for about 25 minutes, until fork-tender but still a little firm.

4. Use a fork to shred the squash flesh into a serving bowl, add the maple syrup, nutmeg, and ginger, and toss to combine.

5. Season with salt and serve.

Per Serving: Calories: 84; Total fat: 2g; Saturated fat: 0g; Sodium: 66mg; Carbohydrates: 17g; Sugar: 10g; Fiber: 2g; Protein: 1g

Roasted Summer Vegetables

GLUTEN-FREE, VEGAN **PREP TIME:** 10 minutes **COOK TIME:** 20 minutes **SERVES** 4

Vegetables get sweeter and deeper in flavor when they are roasted, and this recipe is completely hands-off. What could be simpler? You can also make veggie packets with foil and put them on a grill at medium heat for 15 minutes. Add a couple chicken breasts or a steak to the other side of the grill for a complete dinner.

½ cauliflower head, cut into small florets

½ broccoli head, cut into small florets

2 zucchini, cut into 1-inch chunks

2 yellow bell peppers, seeded and cut into 1-inch chunks

12 asparagus spears, trimmed and cut into 2-inch pieces

1 cup cherry tomatoes

2 tablespoons olive oil

Sea salt

Freshly ground black pepper

1. Preheat the oven to 400°F. Line a baking sheet with parchment paper.

2. In a large bowl, toss the cauliflower, broccoli, zucchini, bell peppers, asparagus, tomatoes, and oil until well mixed.

3. Spread the veggies on the baking sheet and season lightly with salt and pepper.

4. Roast the vegetables for about 20 minutes, stirring occasionally, until the vegetables are tender and lightly caramelized. Serve.

VARIATION: *Any combination of vegetables roasts up beautifully. If you have a little more time, try adding carrots, sweet potatoes, or winter squash to the mixture. Mushrooms, green beans, and pearl onion can be added with no increase in time.*

Per Serving: Calories: 164; Total fat: 8g; Saturated fat: 1g; Sodium: 99mg; Carbohydrates: 21g; Sugar: 7g; Fiber: 7g; Protein: 7g

Broiled Plum Tomatoes
with Goat Cheese

||||||||||||||||||||||||||||||||||||||||||||||||||||||||||||||||||||||||||||||||||||||||

GLUTEN-FREE, VEGETARIAN **PREP TIME:** 10 minutes **COOK TIME:** 10 minutes
SERVES 4

Tomatoes are the ultimate summer choice for salads, sauces, and side dishes. Broiling them creates a pleasing flavor and tasty, lightly caramelized edges. When you add creamy goat cheese and fresh oregano, the dish becomes restaurant worthy. You can use regular tomatoes or halved cherry tomatoes in place of the plum variety; just fill the baking dish in a single layer.

**8 plum tomatoes,
cored and halved
horizontally**

1 tablespoon olive oil

**2 teaspoons
minced garlic**

Sea salt

**Freshly ground
black pepper**

**½ cup crumbled
goat cheese**

**1 tablespoon chopped
fresh oregano**

1. Preheat the oven to broil.

2. Place the tomatoes cut-side down in a 9-by-13-inch baking dish, drizzle with the oil, and sprinkle with the garlic. Season with salt and pepper.

3. Broil the tomatoes for about 6 minutes, until softened and lightly charred.

4. Sprinkle the tomatoes evenly with goat cheese and broil for 4 minutes, until the cheese is melted and lightly browned.

5. Sprinkle with the oregano and serve.

Per Serving: Calories: 92; Total fat: 7g; Saturated fat: 3g; Sodium: 110mg; Carbohydrates: 5g; Sugar: 3g; Fiber: 2g; Protein: 4g

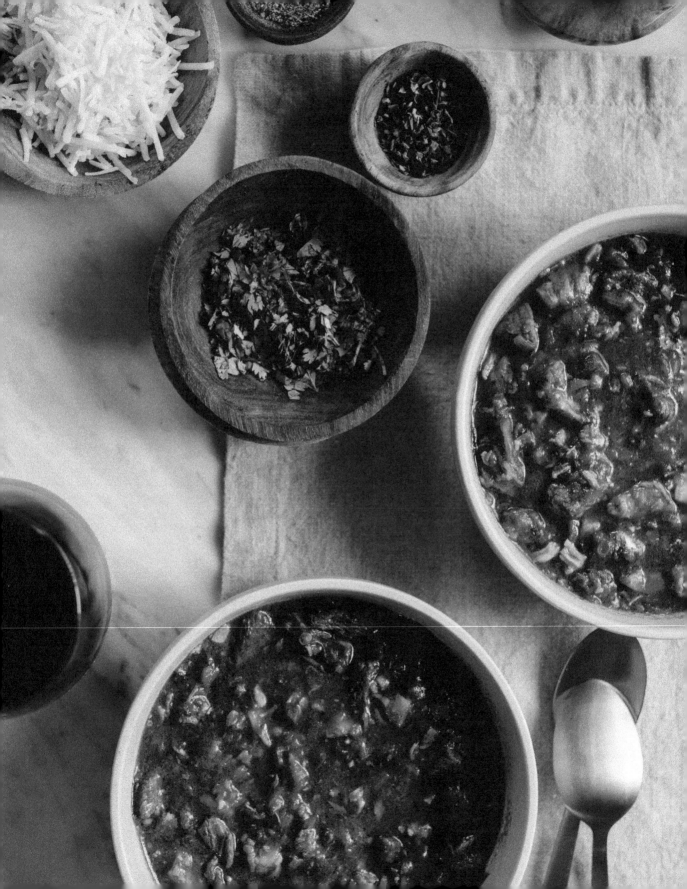

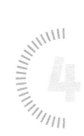

MEAT

Easy Mu Shu Pork

DAIRY-FREE **PREP TIME:** 15 minutes **COOK TIME:** 15 minutes **SERVES** 4

Mu shu pork is a traditional dish in northern China featuring pork, eggs, mushrooms, and daylily buds. This American version omits the eggs and daylily buds and tucks the delicious mixture into tortillas. This recipe is garnished with sesame seeds, which are packed with cholesterol-lowering sterols, protein, fiber, and healthy fats. The combination is heart friendly and can lower blood sugar.

1 tablespoon olive oil

1 pound boneless pork loin chops, thinly sliced

4 cups sliced fresh white mushrooms

2 teaspoons minced garlic

½ small cabbage head, finely shredded

1 red bell pepper, seeded and thinly sliced

2 tablespoons low-sodium soy sauce

1 tablespoon rice vinegar

1 teaspoon toasted sesame oil

1. In a large skillet, heat the olive oil over medium-high heat and sauté the pork for about 6 minutes, until it is just cooked through. Using a slotted spoon, transfer the pork to a plate and set it aside.

2. Add the mushrooms and garlic and sauté for about 5 minutes, until softened and slightly caramelized. Add the cabbage and bell pepper and sauté for about 4 minutes, until tender-crisp.

⅛ teaspoon red pepper flakes

8 (6-inch) whole-wheat tortillas

1 scallion, both white and green parts, thinly sliced on a bias

2 tablespoons sesame seeds

3. Add the pork back to the skillet along with the soy sauce, rice vinegar, sesame oil, and red pepper flakes. Toss to combine and serve scooped into the tortillas and topped with scallions and sesame seeds.

MAKE-AHEAD: *The pork filling is delicious hot or cold and can hold in the refrigerator for up to 3 days. Whip it up for meal prep or when you want a quick grab-and-go meal.*

Per Serving: Calories: 398; Total fat: 14g; Saturated fat: 4g; Sodium: 504mg; Carbohydrates: 38g; Sugar: 6g; Fiber: 10g; Protein: 34g

Skillet Pork Loin with Pears

IIIIIIIIIIIIIIIIIIIIIIIIIIIIIIIIIIIIIIIIIIIIIIIIIIIIIIIIIIIIIIIIIIIIIIIIIIIIIIIIIIIIIIII

DAIRY-FREE, GLUTEN-FREE **PREP TIME:** 10 minutes **COOK TIME:** 18 minutes
SERVES 4

Pork and apples or pears is a classic pairing; the sweetness of the fruit seems to enhance the lightly caramelized meat. Added ginger and thyme creates culinary magic. Pears are low on the glycemic index and high in nutrients and fiber, especially if you leave the skin on.

1 pound boneless pork loin, thinly sliced

Sea salt

Freshly ground black pepper

1 tablespoon olive oil

3 large pears, cored and cut into 1-inch chunks

½ sweet onion, chopped

1 teaspoon peeled and grated fresh ginger

¼ cup unsweetened apple juice

1 teaspoon chopped fresh thyme

1. Season the pork lightly with salt and pepper.

2. In a large skillet, heat the oil over medium-high heat. Sauté the pork for about 6 minutes, until it is browned and just cooked through. Using a slotted spoon, transfer the pork to a plate and set it aside.

3. Add the pears, onion, and ginger and sauté for about 7 minutes, until lightly caramelized. Add the pork back to the skillet along with the apple juice and thyme and simmer for 5 minutes.

4. Serve with your favorite cooked grains or a mixed green salad.

VARIATION: *Try Asian pears, tart apples (if available), or a combination of orchard fruit.*

Per Serving: Calories: 301; Total fat: 8g; Saturated fat: 2g; Sodium: 100mg; Carbohydrates: 31g; Sugar: 18g; Fiber: 7g; Protein: 26g

Pork Fried Brown Rice

DAIRY-FREE **PREP TIME:** 10 minutes **COOK TIME:** 19 minutes **SERVES** 4

Fried rice has a bad reputation as being starchy white rice that's high in fat, but this homemade version uses just a tablespoon of tasty sesame oil and brown rice which slows digestion and keeps you fuller longer. High soluble fiber also means better blood sugar control.

1 tablespoon sesame oil

8 ounces pork tenderloin, cut into ½-inch chunks

4 scallions, both white and green parts, chopped

1 tablespoon peeled and grated fresh ginger

2 teaspoons minced garlic

4 cups cooked (frozen or chilled) brown rice

1 cup frozen or fresh peas

2 tablespoons low-sodium soy sauce

2 large eggs, lightly beaten

1. In a large skillet, heat the oil over medium-high heat. Add the pork and sauté for about 6 minutes, until cooked through. Using a slotted spoon, transfer the pork to a plate and set it aside.

2. Add the scallions, ginger, and garlic and sauté for about 3 minutes, until softened.

3. Add the rice, reserved pork, peas, and soy sauce and sauté for about 10 minutes, until the rice is heated through. Push the rice mixture to the side of the skillet and add the eggs to the empty side.

4. Scramble the eggs and mix them into the fried rice. Serve.

PREP TIP: *Do not use warm rice for this dish. The rice must be completely chilled (or frozen) so it won't fall apart when fried. You can use leftover rice or try the frozen products available in most grocery stores.*

Per Serving: Calories: 388; Total fat: 9g; Saturated fat: 2g; Sodium: 328mg; Carbohydrates: 53g; Sugar: 3g; Fiber: 6g; Protein: 22g

Herbed Pork Cutlets and Roasted Asparagus

|||||||||||||||||||||||||||||||||||||||||||||||||||||||||||||||||||||||||||||||||||||||||||||||

DAIRY-FREE, GLUTEN-FREE **PREP TIME:** 10 minutes, plus 30 minutes optional marinating time **COOK TIME:** 10 minutes **SERVES** 4

Pork chops are enhanced by whatever spices or herbs you serve with them, such as bright, fresh cilantro and parsley. Asparagus is very high in folate, and you'll get about 50 percent of your recommended daily value in this serving size. Folate can help lower the risk of heart disease, which can be a concern for people with type 2 diabetes.

2 tablespoons plus 1 teaspoon olive oil, divided

Juice of 2 limes, divided

1 tablespoon chopped fresh cilantro

1 tablespoon chopped fresh parsley

2 teaspoons minced garlic

4 (4-ounce) boneless center cut pork chops, pounded to ¼-inch thick

Sea salt

1. In a large bowl, combine 2 tablespoons of the oil, the juice from 1 lime, the cilantro, parsley, and garlic until well mixed. Add the pork and toss to coat. Season lightly with salt and pepper. Let it rest 30 minutes at room temperature if you have set aside additional time to marinate.

2. Preheat the oven to broil and set the rack in the middle.

3. Heat a large skillet over medium-high heat and fry the pork chops for about 8 minutes in total, turning halfway through, until just cooked through and still juicy.

Freshly ground black pepper

3 asparagus bunches (about 36 stalks), woody ends trimmed

4. While the pork chops are cooking, arrange the asparagus on a baking sheet, drizzle with the remaining 1 teaspoon of olive oil, and season with salt and pepper. Broil for about 2 minutes, until tender. Remove and drizzle with the remaining lime juice.

5. Serve each pork chop with a portion of asparagus.

Per Serving: Calories: 201; Total fat: 6g; Saturated fat: 2g; Sodium: 95mg; Carbohydrates: 11g; Sugar: 4g; Fiber: 5g; Protein: 28g

Sesame Pork Lettuce Wraps

DAIRY-FREE, GLUTEN-FREE **PREP TIME:** 13 minutes **COOK TIME:** 17 minutes
SERVES 4

Who doesn't like a savory, spiced filling tucked into tender lettuce leaves? Lettuce wraps are a popular street food in Southeast Asia and other parts of the world. The bean sprouts in this version are more than just bulk; they are very high in antioxidants and contain heart-friendly soluble fiber. Including sprouts regularly in your diet can help lower blood sugar and cholesterol.

1 tablespoon
sesame oil

12 ounces
ground pork

2 cups bean sprouts

1 red bell pepper,
seeded and chopped

2 scallions, both
white and green
parts, chopped

⅛ teaspoon red
pepper flakes

8 butter or iceberg
lettuce leaves

Sesame seeds,
for garnish

Lime wedges,
for garnish

1. In a large skillet, heat the oil over medium-high heat. Sauté the pork for about 7 minutes, until it is cooked through.

2. Add the bean sprouts, bell pepper, and scallions and sauté for about 10 minutes, until softened.

3. Add the red pepper flakes and toss to mix.

4. Scoop the mixture evenly among the lettuce leaves and serve topped with sesame seeds, with lime wedges on the side.

Per Serving: Calories: 296; Total fat: 20g; Saturated fat: 6g; Sodium: 57mg; Carbohydrates: 8g; Sugar: 2g; Fiber: 3g; Protein: 20g

Pork and Cabbage Stir-Fry

DAIRY-FREE **PREP TIME:** 15 minutes **COOK TIME:** 13 minutes **SERVES** 4

Stir-fries don't have to be complicated to be delicious. Lean pork loin, cabbage, and carrots are elevated by the peanut butter sauce in this dish. You might end up eating it with a spoon! Peanut butter can keep you satiated for hours and is packed with blood sugar–lowering monounsaturated fats. Opt for a natural peanut butter containing just peanuts or peanuts and salt.

Juice of 2 limes

2 tablespoons all-natural peanut butter

1 tablespoon honey

2 teaspoons low-sodium soy sauce

1 tablespoon sesame oil

1 pound pork loin center cut chops, thinly sliced

½ small head cabbage, finely shredded

2 carrots, shredded

½ onion, thinly sliced

2 teaspoons minced garlic

1. In a small bowl, stir together the lime juice, peanut butter, honey, and soy sauce until well combined. Set it aside.

2. In a large skillet, heat the oil over medium-high heat and sauté the pork for about 6 minutes, until browned and just cooked through. Using a slotted spoon, transfer the pork to a plate and set aside.

3. Add the cabbage, carrots, onion, and garlic and sauté for about 6 minutes, until the vegetables are tender-crisp.

4. Add the pork and sauce to the skillet and toss to heat through, about 1 minute. Serve.

VARIATION: *Try making the sauce with almond or cashew butter for a slightly different, but still delightful, flavor.*

Per Serving: Calories: 329; Total fat: 15g; Saturated fat: 4g; Sodium: 199mg; Carbohydrates: 22g; Sugar: 12g; Fiber: 7g; Protein: 29g

Roasted Spice-Rubbed Pork Tenderloin

DAIRY-FREE, GLUTEN-FREE **PREP TIME:** 5 minutes, plus 10 minutes resting time
COOK TIME: 15 minutes **SERVES** 4

Warm spices create a gorgeous autumn-inspired roasted pork tenderloin that tastes like it belongs in a fine-dining restaurant. Cinnamon is an excellent rub choice because it may help lower blood sugar by increasing insulin sensitivity. This effect can last for up to 12 hours after eating this spice. Try serving the pork with Roasted Summer Vegetables (page 57) or Maple Spaghetti Squash (page 56).

1 teaspoon ground cinnamon

½ teaspoon ground cumin

½ teaspoon ground coriander

¼ teaspoon paprika

¼ teaspoon garlic powder

¼ teaspoon ground ginger

1 (1-pound) pork tenderloin

2 teaspoons olive oil

1. In a small bowl, combine the cinnamon, cumin, coriander, paprika, garlic powder, and ginger.

2. Rub the spice mixture generously all over the pork.

3. In a large skillet, heat the oil over medium-high heat. Cook the tenderloin for about 15 minutes, until it is browned on all sides and just cooked through.

4. Rest the meat on a cutting board for 10 minutes before slicing. Serve.

Per Serving: Calories: 147; Total fat: 5g; Saturated fat: 1g; Sodium: 61mg; Carbohydrates: 1g; Sugar: 0g; Fiber: 0g; Protein: 24g

Pork Piccata

DAIRY-FREE **PREP TIME:** 15 minutes **COOK TIME:** 15 minutes **SERVES** 4

Piccata is an Italian dish traditionally prepared with veal. This pork version is equally tender and satisfying. Piccata means "to pound flat" in Italian, and you can do that here with a mallet or rolling pin, or buy the pork pre-pounded. Eating lean meat at least a few times a week can help maintain muscle mass and keep you feeling full.

½ cup whole-wheat flour or almond flour

½ teaspoon garlic powder

¼ teaspoon sea salt

¼ teaspoon freshly ground black pepper

4 (4-ounce) boneless pork chops, pounded flat

2 teaspoons olive oil

½ cup low-sodium chicken broth

Juice and zest of 1 lemon, divided

2 tablespoons capers

1 tablespoon chopped fresh parsley

1. In a small bowl, combine the flour, garlic powder, salt, and pepper. Dredge the pork chops in the flour mixture, shaking off any excess.

2. In a large skillet, heat the oil over medium-high heat. Cook the pork, turning once, until browned and just cooked through, about 10 minutes. Transfer the pork to a plate and set aside.

3. Add the broth to the skillet, scraping up any browned bits. Add the lemon juice, reduce the heat to low, and simmer for about 2 minutes, until it is reduced by half.

4. Add the lemon zest, capers, and parsley.

5. Serve the pork cutlets with the lemon-caper sauce.

Per Serving: Calories: 220; Total fat: 7g; Saturated fat: 2g; Sodium: 303mg; Carbohydrates: 12g; Sugar: 0g; Fiber: 2g; Protein: 28g

Mongolian-Inspired Beef

DAIRY-FREE **PREP TIME:** 12 minutes **COOK TIME:** 18 minutes **SERVES** 4

This dish is a takeout favorite that is just as easy to make at home. This version might not be as sweet as your favorite restaurant order but makes for a healthier choice. The edamame adds a gorgeous bright accent to the darker beef and soy-spiked sauce. Edamame contains just over 10 grams of fiber per cup, so it is fabulous for regulating blood sugar and reducing the risk of heart disease. This legume is also very high in protein, so it contributes to keeping you feeling full longer after this meal.

3 teaspoons olive oil, divided

1 tablespoon minced garlic

1 teaspoon peeled and grated fresh ginger

¼ cup water

2 tablespoons low-sodium soy sauce

2 tablespoons maple syrup

⅛ teaspoon red pepper flakes

1 pound flank steak, cut into thin strips

1. In a small saucepan, heat 1 teaspoon of the oil over medium heat and sauté the garlic and ginger for about 2 minutes, until softened. Stir in the water, soy sauce, maple syrup, and red pepper flakes, and bring to a boil. Reduce the heat to low and simmer for 2 minutes. Remove the saucepan from the heat and set aside.

2. Place the flank steak strips in a large plastic freezer bag and add the cornstarch. Toss to coat the pieces.

¼ cup cornstarch

**2 cups
shelled edamame**

**1 red bell pepper,
seeded and
thinly sliced**

**2 scallions, both
white and green
parts, chopped**

3. In a large skillet, heat the remaining
   2 teaspoons of oil over medium-high heat
   and, working in three batches, sauté the
   steak until lightly browned but still slightly
   pink, about 2 minutes a batch. Using a
   slotted spoon, transfer the steak to a plate
   and set aside.

4. Add the edamame, bell pepper, and scallions and sauté for about 4 minutes,
   until softened. Add the steak and sauce
   back to the skillet and toss for about
   2 minutes, until well mixed and heated
   through. Serve.

PREP TIP: *Frozen edamame is found in most grocery
stores. Look for a shelled product that is flash frozen for
the best quality and run it under warm water for a couple
of minutes before adding to the skillet.*

Per Serving: Calories: 355; Total fat: 12g; Saturated fat: 3g;
Sodium: 325mg; Carbohydrates: 25g; Sugar: 9g; Fiber: 5g;
Protein: 34g

Beefy Taco Skillet

GLUTEN-FREE **PREP TIME:** 10 minutes **COOK TIME:** 20 minutes **SERVES** 4

Instead of stuffing spicy beef filling into shells, this easy recipe combines all the elements of the perfect taco in a tasty one-pot meal. The added onion in this dish is not just for flavor; it contains an insoluble fiber that increases the levels of a blood sugar–lowering hormone called ghrelin.

1 teaspoon olive oil

8 ounces 93 percent lean ground beef

1 onion, chopped

1 green bell pepper, chopped

1 (15-ounce) can low-sodium black beans, drained and rinsed

1 (15-ounce) can no-salt-added diced tomatoes, drained

2 tablespoons low-sodium taco seasoning

4 (6-inch) corn tortillas, cut into 1-inch pieces

½ cup shredded low-fat Cheddar cheese

1 cup shredded lettuce

1. In a large skillet, heat the oil over medium-high heat and sauté the beef until it is cooked through, about 6 minutes. Add the onion and bell pepper and sauté for about 4 minutes, until softened.

2. Add the black beans, tomatoes, and taco seasoning and bring to a simmer. Reduce the heat and simmer for 6 minutes. Add the tortillas and cheese and stir for about 4 minutes, until the tortillas soften.

3. Serve topped with shredded lettuce and additional cheese, if desired.

PREP TIP: *If you have a little extra time, you can also bake this casserole-style dish at 350°F for 40 minutes. Just combine everything after the first step and pop the covered skillet in the oven.*

Per Serving: Calories: 320; Total fat: 10g; Saturated fat: 4g; Sodium: 251mg; Carbohydrates: 36g; Sugar: 5g; Fiber: 10g; Protein: 24g

Classic Beef Hamburgers

DAIRY-FREE **PREP TIME:** 10 minutes **COOK TIME:** 15 minutes **SERVES** 4

Burgers are a favorite choice because they are easy to make at home and taste incredible. This is a beef-based recipe, but you could use half pork. Look for no-sugar-added high-fiber whole-grain buns to help manage blood sugar levels.

1 teaspoon olive oil

½ cup chopped onion

2 teaspoons minced garlic

1 pound 93 percent lean ground beef

½ cup whole-wheat bread crumbs

1 large egg

1 teaspoon chopped fresh parsley

¼ teaspoon sea salt

⅛ teaspoon freshly ground black pepper

4 whole-grain hamburger buns

Optional toppings

Cheese

Lettuce

Tomatoes

1. In a small skillet, heat the oil over medium-high heat and sauté the onion and garlic for about 3 minutes, until softened.

2. In a large bowl, mix the cooked veggies, ground beef, bread crumbs, egg, parsley, salt, and pepper until well combined.

3. Divide the mixture into 4 equal portions and form into ½-inch-thick patties.

4. Preheat a grill to medium-high and grill the burgers for 5 to 6 minutes per side, turning halfway through, until cooked through.

5. Serve on buns with desired toppings.

PREP TIP: *You can cook the burgers in a large skillet over medium-high heat for 5 minutes on each a side.*

Per Serving: Calories: 368; Total fat: 15g; Saturated fat: 4g; Sodium: 368mg; Carbohydrates: 25g; Sugar: 4g; Fiber: 4g; Protein: 32g

Spicy Beef Chili

GLUTEN-FREE PREP TIME: 10 minutes **COOK TIME:** 20 minutes **SERVES** 4

People take pride in their chili; recipes are handed down through generations, and many include secret ingredients like coffee and chocolate. This is a simple version: lean beef, veggies, heaps of beans, and a generous amount of chili powder. Of course, you can jazz it up with your own favorite additions. Keep in mind this recipe is speedy, but chili often tastes better the next day.

2 teaspoons olive oil

12 ounces 93 percent lean ground beef

1 onion, chopped

1 green bell pepper, seeded and chopped

2 teaspoons minced garlic

1 (28-ounce) can no-salt-added diced tomatoes, drained

1 (15-ounce) can low-sodium black beans, drained and rinsed

1 (15-ounce) can low-sodium cannellini beans, drained

2 tablespoons chili powder

Sour cream, for garnish (optional)

1. In a large saucepan, heat the oil over medium-high heat and sauté the ground beef for about 6 minutes, until it is cooked through. Add the onion, bell pepper, and garlic and sauté for about 4 minutes, until softened.

2. Add the tomatoes, black beans, cannellini beans, and chili powder and simmer for 10 minutes.

3. Serve topped with sour cream (if using).

PREP TIP: *You can make this in a slow cooker by adding all the ingredients and ¼ cup of water to the insert and cooking on high for 3 to 4 hours.*

Per Serving: Calories: 418; Total fat: 9g; Saturated fat: 2g; Sodium: 195mg; Carbohydrates: 54g; Sugar: 7g; Fiber: 20g; Protein: 36g

Sloppy Joes

DAIRY-FREE **PREP TIME:** 10 minutes **COOK TIME:** 20 minutes **SERVES** 4

Sloppy Joes were a staple growing up, but we used canned sauce and bread slices. This recipe has a rich, thick home-made sauce with yummy lentils. Lentils are very high in resistant starch, a carb that passes through your system undigested, so impacts blood sugar minimally. This gut-friendly starch also feeds the healthy bacteria found in your digestive tract.

1 teaspoon olive oil

8 ounces 93 percent lean ground beef

¼ onion, chopped

1 teaspoon minced garlic

1 cup no-salt-added tomato sauce

½ cup canned lentils, drained and rinsed

2 tablespoons no-salt-added tomato paste

1 teaspoon brown sugar

¼ teaspoon chili powder

¼ teaspoon dry mustard

Sea salt

4 whole-grain buns, halved

1. In a large skillet, heat the oil over medium-high heat. Add the beef and cook for about 6 minutes, until the beef is no longer pink. Add the onion and garlic and sauté for 4 minutes.

2. Add the tomato sauce, lentils, tomato paste, brown sugar, chili powder, mustard, and salt. Cover, reduce the heat to low, and simmer the mixture for 10 minutes.

3. Divide the sloppy joe mixture among the buns and serve.

Per Serving: Calories: 257; Total fat: 6g; Saturated fat: 2g; Sodium: 295mg; Carbohydrates: 31g; Sugar: 7g; Fiber: 5g; Protein: 20g

Sheet-Pan Steak and Broccoli

DAIRY-FREE, GLUTEN-FREE **PREP TIME:** 15 minutes **COOK TIME:** 10 minutes
SERVES 4

Sheet-pan recipes are my favorite no-fuss or mess meals;
Broccoli is a welcome addition to a sheet pan because it
roasts up tender, and its flavor deepens as it cooks. In addi-
tion, broccoli is packed with fiber, vitamin C, magnesium, and
chromium, which can help reduce blood glucose levels and
control blood sugar long-term.

2 (8-ounce) sirloin steaks, about 1-inch thick, trimmed of visible fat

1 tablespoon olive oil, divided

Sea salt

Freshly ground black pepper

2 broccoli heads, cut into florets

1. Preheat the oven to 450°F. Line a baking sheet with foil.

2. Cover the steaks with 1 teaspoon of oil and season all over with salt and pepper.

3. Place the steaks on one-third of the baking sheet.

4. In a large bowl, toss the broccoli, onion, and remaining 2 teaspoons of oil. Season lightly with salt and pepper.

5. Spread the vegetables on the other two-thirds of the baking sheet.

1 small red onion, thinly sliced

Juice of 1 lemon

6. Roast the steaks and vegetables, turning once, about 4 minutes per side for medium-rare, until the steaks are browned and have reached the desired doneness.

7. Let the steaks rest for 10 minutes and slice thinly on a bias against the grain. Drizzle the broccoli with the lemon juice. Serve.

Per Serving: Calories: 296; Total fat: 10g; Saturated fat: 3g; Sodium: 205mg; Carbohydrates: 23g; Sugar: 6g; Fiber: 8g; Protein: 33g

Beef Tomato Ragù

IIIIIIIIIIIIIIIIIIIIIIIIIIIIIIIIIIIIIIIIIIIIIIIIIIIIIIIIIIIIIIIIIIIIIIIIIIIIIIIIIIIII

DAIRY-FREE PREP TIME: 10 minutes **COOK TIME:** 20 minutes **SERVES** 4

Everyone needs a simple, foolproof pasta sauce, and this might be the one you come back to again and again. It is flavored generously with garlic, onions, and fresh herbs and can be the base of a lasagna or spooned over any favorite pasta shape.

8 ounces whole-grain spaghetti

1 tablespoon olive oil

12 ounces 93 percent lean ground beef

1 onion, chopped

1 tablespoon minced garlic

1 (28-ounce) can no-salt-added diced tomatoes

2 tablespoons chopped fresh basil, or 2 teaspoons dried basil

1 tablespoon chopped fresh oregano, or 1 teaspoon dried oregano

Sea salt

Freshly ground black pepper

1. Bring a large saucepan filled three-quarters full of water to a boil over high heat. Add the spaghetti, reduce the heat to medium-low, and simmer until al dente, about 18 minutes. Drain and set aside.

2. While the spaghetti is cooking, in a large skillet, heat the oil over medium-high heat. Add the beef and brown it for about 6 minutes, or until cooked through.

3. Add the onion and garlic and sauté for about 3 minutes, until softened.

4. Stir in the tomatoes and their juices, basil, and oregano and bring the mixture to a boil. Reduce the heat to low and simmer for about 10 minutes.

5. Season the sauce with salt and pepper and serve over the cooked pasta.

Per Serving: Calories: 385; Total fat: 9g; Saturated fat: 3g; Sodium: 82mg; Carbohydrates: 52g; Sugar: 6g; Fiber: 9g; Protein: 29g

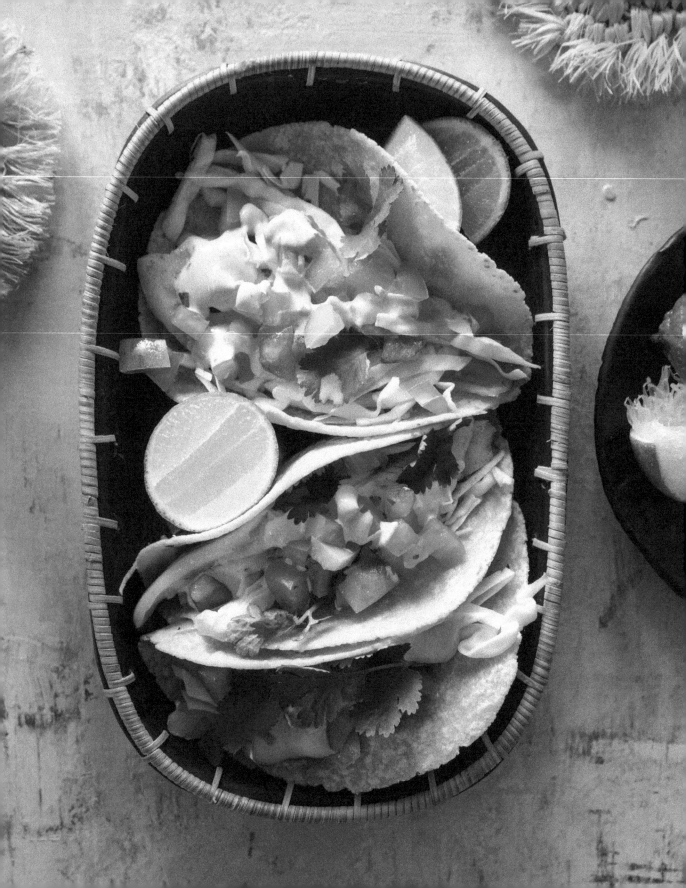

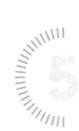

POULTRY AND SEAFOOD

Sheet-Pan Chicken Parmesan with Cauliflower

GLUTEN-FREE **PREP TIME:** 10 minutes **COOK TIME:** 20 minutes **SERVES** 4

This is a deconstructed chicken Parmesan that uses fresh ingredients and does not bread the chicken. It pairs well with the simple roasted cauliflower that shares the sheet pan. Cauliflower is an excellent choice for a type 2 diabetes diet because it contains sulforaphane, like all cruciferous vegetables. This compound can lower the risk of cardiovascular disease by lowering oxidative stress, a contributor to heart disease.

1 cauliflower head, cut into small florets

1 tablespoon olive oil

Sea salt

Freshly ground black pepper

4 (4-ounce) boneless, skinless chicken breasts, pounded to ½-inch thick

2 tomatoes, sliced

1. Preheat the oven to 400°F. Line a baking sheet with parchment paper.

2. In a medium bowl, toss the cauliflower and oil until well coated and season with salt and pepper. Spread the cauliflower on half the baking sheet.

3. Lightly season the chicken breasts with salt and pepper.

4. Place the chicken on the empty side of the baking sheet and top each with the tomato slices and Parmesan cheese.

**½ cup grated
Parmesan cheese**

**1 tablespoon chopped
fresh basil**

5. Bake for about 20 minutes, or until the chicken is just cooked through and the vegetables are tender.

6. Serve topped with basil.

VARIATION: *You can swap out the sliced tomatoes for your favorite store-bought low-sugar marinara sauce if you want a more traditional version.*

Per Serving: Calories: 287; Total fat: 10g; Saturated fat: 3g; Sodium: 383mg; Carbohydrates: 16g; Sugar: 6g; Fiber: 5g; Protein: 33g

Creamy Coconut Chicken Soup

DAIRY-FREE, GLUTEN-FREE **PREP TIME:** 10 minutes **COOK TIME:** 20 minutes
SERVES 4

A lovely restaurant inspired this recipe for creamy and luscious coconut chicken soup. You can also make it without the chicken and just add extra veggies or chickpeas. However, the chicken does add a comforting flavor, and the lean protein is highly satiating. If you have leftover chicken or turkey from another recipe, it can be thrown in here, too.

1 tablespoon coconut oil

1 onion, chopped

1 red bell pepper, seeded and chopped

2 teaspoons minced garlic

2 teaspoons peeled and grated fresh ginger

3 cups low-sodium chicken broth

1 (13½-ounce) can light coconut milk

1 sweet potato, peeled and chopped

2 cups chopped cooked store-bought rotisserie chicken

1 lime

1. In a large stockpot, heat the oil over medium-high heat and sauté the onion, bell pepper, garlic, and ginger for about 5 minutes, until softened.

2. Add the broth, coconut milk, sweet potato, chicken, lime juice, and lime zest and bring to a boil. Reduce the heat to low and simmer for 15 minutes, until the sweet potatoes are tender.

3. Serve hot.

VARIATION: *For a lovely finish, top the soup with chopped fresh cilantro.*

Per Serving: Calories: 347; Total fat: 19g; Saturated fat: 12g; Sodium: 142mg; Carbohydrates: 18g; Sugar: 4g; Fiber: 3g; Protein: 26g

Shawarma Chicken with Chickpeas and Sweet Potato

DAIRY-FREE, GLUTEN-FREE **PREP TIME:** 10 minutes **COOK TIME:** 20 minutes
SERVES 4

Shawarma often refers to the cooking method—strips of seasoned meat stacked in a cone shape and slow-roasted on a rotisserie—but here, it refers to the spices used in the dish. Chickpeas add fiber and B vitamins, and they are very low on the glycemic index—perfect for type 2 diabetes management.

1 (15-ounce) can low-sodium chickpeas, drained and rinsed

1 sweet potato, peeled and cut into ½-inch chunks

1 tablespoon olive oil

4 teaspoons store-bought shawarma spice, divided

1 pound boneless, skinless chicken breast, cut into 1-inch chunks

1. Preheat the oven to 400°F. Line a baking sheet with parchment paper.

2. In a medium bowl, toss the chickpeas, sweet potato, oil, and 1 teaspoon shawarma spice until well combined. Spread the mixture on half of the baking sheet.

3. Add the chicken breast to the bowl and toss with the remaining 3 teaspoons of shawarma spice. Spread the chicken chunks on the other half of the baking sheet.

4. Bake for about 20 minutes, tossing halfway through, until the chicken is cooked through. Serve.

VARIATION: *You can tuck the chicken, chickpeas, and sweet potato into a pita for lunch the next day.*

Per Serving: Calories: 260; Total fat: 7g; Saturated fat: 1g; Sodium: 235mg; Carbohydrates: 20g; Sugar: 4g; Fiber: 5g; Protein: 30g

Chicken Salad Pitas

PREP TIME: 25 minutes **SERVES** 4

I make many versions of chicken salad because this tasty protein goes well with both savory and sweet ingredients. You will find both here with the apple, veggies, tart yogurt, and crunch of cashews. Low-calorie, high-fiber apples can control blood sugar spikes and help lower bad cholesterol. The nutty topping is also fiber-rich and a healthy protein source.

2 cups diced cooked store-bought rotisserie chicken breast

½ cup chopped celery

½ cup shredded carrot

1 apple, cored and chopped

1 scallion, both white and green parts, chopped

¼ cup low-fat plain Greek yogurt

2 tablespoons chopped cashews

Pinch sea salt

Pinch freshly ground black pepper

4 (6-inch) whole-wheat pitas, halved

1 cup shredded lettuce

1. In a large bowl, mix the chicken, celery, carrot, apple, scallion, yogurt, cashews, salt, and pepper until well combined.

2. Spoon the chicken mixture into the pita halves, top with lettuce, and serve 2 halves per person.

VARIATION: *Whole-grain tortillas or large lettuce leaves make delicious containers for the creamy filling if pita bread is unavailable.*

Per Serving: Calories: 254; Total fat: 6g; Saturated fat: 1g; Sodium: 233mg; Carbohydrates: 27g; Sugar: 7g; Fiber: 4g; Protein: 24g

Roasted Chicken with Tzatziki

GLUTEN-FREE **PREP TIME:** 6 minutes **COOK TIME:** 24 minutes **SERVES** 4

Simple roasted chicken is a culinary delight, especially when topped with this cool, creamy sauce. The chicken here is lightly seasoned with paprika for a lovely golden color and fragrant thyme. You can get a nice store-bought tzatziki, but why not make your own, so the ingredients are exactly what you want? Low-fat Greek yogurt is a must for taste and nutrition reasons. The combination of protein, carbs, and probiotics can help reduce the risk of heart disease, control hunger, and lower blood sugar levels.

4 (4-ounce) boneless, skinless chicken breasts

Sea salt

Freshly ground black pepper

1 teaspoon chopped fresh thyme, or ½ teaspoon dried thyme

¼ teaspoon paprika

1 tablespoon olive oil

½ cup Tzatziki Sauce (page 127), or store-bought

1. Preheat the oven to 400°F.

2. Lightly season the chicken breasts with salt and pepper, then cover them in the thyme and paprika.

3. In a large ovenproof skillet, heat the oil over medium-high heat. Brown the chicken breasts on both sides for about 4 minutes in total, turning halfway through.

4. Place the skillet in the oven and roast for about 20 minutes, until cooked through.

5. Serve the chicken breasts topped with tzatziki.

Per Serving: Calories: 192; Total fat: 7g; Saturated fat: 1g; Sodium: 112mg; Carbohydrates: 5g; Sugar: 3g; Fiber: 1g; Protein: 27g

Turkey Taco Stuffed Sweet Potatoes

GLUTEN-FREE **PREP TIME:** 15 minutes **COOK TIME:** 15 minutes **SERVES** 2

When I worked in North Africa as a chef, I discovered the most delicious stuffed potatoes in the world called kumpir. Everything you could think of was used as a topping. This version of that incredible dish features sweet potatoes instead because they are packed with soluble fiber and nutrients including carotenoids. This combination can help reduce insulin resistance and slow digestion.

2 medium sweet potatoes, scrubbed and pricked with a fork

8 ounces ground turkey

2 tablespoons water

1 tablespoon low-sodium taco seasoning

¼ cup store-bought salsa

¼ cup shredded Cheddar cheese

1. Microwave the sweet potatoes for about 10 minutes, until soft.

2. While the potatoes are cooking, sauté the turkey for about 10 minutes, until cooked through. Add the water and taco seasoning and cook for 3 minutes.

3. Preheat the oven to broil.

4. Cut the sweet potatoes in half lengthwise and press them open. Scoop the turkey filling into the potatoes and top with the salsa and cheese.

Optional toppings

Sliced avocado

Jalapeño peppers

Low-fat sour cream

Sliced olives

5. Place the sweet potatoes in an 8-inch baking dish and broil for about 2 minutes, until the cheese is melted.

6. Serve with additional toppings (if using).

MAKE-AHEAD: *You can also bake the sweet pota-toes ahead in a 400°F oven (after pricking them) for 40 minutes. Then take them from the refrigerator, warm them in a 300°F oven while cooking the spiced meat, stuff, and broil.*

Per Serving: Calories: 467; Total fat: 13g; Saturated fat: 5g; Sodium: 324mg; Carbohydrates: 55g; Sugar: 7g; Fiber: 7g; Protein: 30g

Turkey Meatballs

DAIRY-FREE, GLUTEN-FREE **PREP TIME:** 10 minutes **COOK TIME:** 20 minutes
SERVES 4

This tasty, simple recipe is the base for many meals in my house and in some of the restaurants I have worked in over the years. I throw the meatballs onto pasta, stuff them into pitas, or add heaps of fiber-rich veggies to the sheet pan for a complete meal. You can add other seasonings, such as herbs, ginger, or even a splash of soy sauce, for your own unique spin.

1 pound lean ground turkey

¼ cup almond flour or whole-wheat bread crumbs

¼ cup chopped onion

1 large egg

1 teaspoon minced garlic

½ teaspoon chopped fresh thyme

¼ teaspoon sea salt

⅛ teaspoon ground nutmeg

⅛ teaspoon freshly ground black pepper

1. Preheat the oven to 400°F. Line a baking sheet with parchment paper.

2. In a large bowl, mix the turkey, almond flour, onion, egg, garlic, thyme, salt, nutmeg, and pepper. Form the mixture into 1-inch meatballs.

3. Bake for about 20 minutes, turning halfway through, until cooked through and browned.

4. Serve with Quinoa with Chopped Pistachios (page 54) or Roasted Summer Vegetables (page 57).

VARIATION: *Try ground chicken, beef, or pork, depending on your preference. The cooking time will not change.*

Per Serving: Calories: 228; Total fat: 13g; Saturated fat: 3g; Sodium: 174mg; Carbohydrates: 3g; Sugar: 1g; Fiber: 1g; Protein: 24g

Speedy Fish Stew

DAIRY-FREE, GLUTEN-FREE **PREP TIME:** 10 minutes **COOK TIME:** 20 minutes
SERVES 4

I learned to appreciate fish stew when working in Libya, where the fresh seafood still glistening with seawater when coming through my kitchen door. This speedy stew has tons of fiber-rich veggies, lentils, and chunks of fresh salmon. Fatty fish like salmon are high in omega-3 fatty acids, which can cut the risk of stroke and heart disease.

1 tablespoon olive oil

1 red bell pepper, seeded and chopped

1 onion, chopped

3 celery stalks, chopped

1 tablespoon minced garlic

2 teaspoons ground cumin

6 cups low-sodium vegetable broth

1 (15-ounce) can no-salt-added diced tomatoes

1 (15-ounce) can low-sodium lentils, drained and rinsed

12 ounces salmon, cubed

Freshly ground black pepper

1. In a large stockpot, heat the oil over medium-high heat.

2. Sauté the bell pepper, onion, celery, garlic, and cumin for about 4 minutes until softened.

3. Stir in the broth, tomatoes and their juices, and lentils and bring to a boil. Reduce the heat to medium-low and simmer for 10 minutes.

4. Add the fish and simmer for about 6 minutes, until just cooked through. Season with pepper and serve.

VARIATION: *Try any firm fish for this stew, such as halibut, haddock, or trout, as well as shrimp or scallops, if available.*

Per Serving: Calories: 396; Total fat: 16g; Saturated fat: 3g; Sodium: 357mg; Carbohydrates: 40g; Sugar: 16g; Fiber: 12g; Protein: 24g

Baked Almond Shrimp with Grapefruit Salsa

DAIRY-FREE, GLUTEN-FREE **PREP TIME:** 20 minutes **COOK TIME:** 10 minutes
SERVES 4

This recipe is gorgeous; it is a feast for the eyes with its festive colors. Grapefruit can improve insulin sensitivity and lower blood sugar, so include the juice when you cut the fruit. Shrimp contains cholesterol but is still a healthy option in moderation and when prepared with a light coating of almonds.

For the salsa

2 ruby red grapefruits, peeled and chopped

½ cucumber, chopped

½ yellow bell pepper, seeded and chopped

1 teaspoon chopped fresh cilantro

Sea salt

For the shrimp

Nonstick cooking spray

1 pound (21 to 25 count) raw shrimp, peeled and deveined

2 large eggs, beaten

1 cup almond flour

To make the salsa

1. In a small bowl, mix the grapefruit, cucumber, bell pepper, and cilantro. Season with salt and set it aside.

To make the shrimp

2. Preheat the oven to 450°F. Lightly coat a baking sheet with cooking spray.

3. Dredge the shrimp in the egg and then the almond flour until well coated.

4. Place the shrimp on the baking sheet and bake for about 10 minutes, until cooked through and the coating is golden brown.

5. Serve the shrimp with grapefruit salsa.

Per Serving: Calories: 232; Total fat: 8g; Saturated fat: 1g; Sodium: 193mg; Carbohydrates: 16g; Sugar: 1g; Fiber: 4g; Protein: 28g

Coconut-Turmeric Baked Tilapia and Quinoa

DAIRY-FREE, GLUTEN-FREE **PREP TIME:** 5 minutes **COOK TIME:** 25 minutes
SERVES 4

Fish—and grains—baked in coconut milk become tender, and the rich flavor infuses the other ingredients. The added tomatoes, herbs, and spices boost the taste and, in the case of turmeric, creates a luscious golden hue. Turmeric contains curcumin, which can help lower blood sugar and reduce inflammation. Don't omit the black pepper because it activates the curcumin.

1 cup quinoa, rinsed

1 cup low-sodium chicken broth

1 cup light coconut milk

1 tomato, chopped

2 teaspoons minced garlic

1 teaspoon ground turmeric

⅛ teaspoon freshly ground black pepper

1 pound tilapia fillets

2 tablespoons chopped fresh cilantro, for garnish

1. Preheat the oven to 400°F.

2. Combine the quinoa, chicken broth, coconut milk, tomato, garlic, turmeric, and pepper in a deep 9-inch square baking or casserole dish.

3. Nestle the fish in the quinoa mixture and cover the baking dish with foil.

4. Bake for about 25 minutes, until the quinoa is tender and the fish is cooked through. Top with cilantro and serve.

VARIATION: *Any fish works here, such as cod, sole, or halibut. The cooking time shouldn't change unless your fish is over 1 inch thick.*

Per Serving: Calories: 343; Total fat: 11g; Saturated fat: 6g; Sodium: 86mg; Carbohydrates: 31g; Sugar: 1g; Fiber: 5g; Protein: 31g

Lemon Trout with Garlic Potato Hash Browns

DAIRY-FREE, GLUTEN-FREE **PREP TIME:** 10 minutes **COOK TIME:** 20 minutes
SERVES 4

I live in northern Canada, where there are sparkling lakes around every corner of the road and fishing is a way of life. This recipe is inspired by countless shore lunches over five decades. Eating fish even once a week can reduce the risk of cardio-vascular disease—one of the most serious complications of diabetes—by 40 percent. Trout is a fatty fish, so it offers some extra protection, although any fish can be used here.

2 large russet potatoes, chopped

¼ onion, chopped

2 teaspoons minced garlic

½ teaspoon smoked paprika

2 tablespoons olive oil, divided

Sea salt

Freshly ground black pepper

1. Preheat the oven to 400°F. Line a baking sheet with parchment paper.

2. In a large bowl, toss the potatoes, onion, garlic, paprika, and 1 tablespoon of the oil. Spread the potatoes on half the baking sheet and season lightly with salt and pepper.

3. Place the fish on the other half of the baking sheet, brush with the remaining 1 tablespoon of oil, and season with salt and pepper.

4 (4-ounce) boneless, skinless trout fillets

1 tablespoon chopped fresh parsley

1 lemon, quartered

4. Bake for about 20 minutes, tossing halfway through, until the potatoes are golden and lightly crispy and the fish is flaky.

5. Serve topped with parsley and lemon wedges.

VARIATION: *If you don't want to use regular potatoes, use any root vegetable, such as carrots, sweet potatoes, parsnips, or winter squash.*

Per Serving: Calories: 349; Total fat: 10g; Saturated fat: 2g; Sodium: 85mg; Carbohydrates: 35g; Sugar: 2g; Fiber: 3g; Protein: 27g

Sesame Salmon with Bok Choy

DAIRY-FREE, GLUTEN-FREE **PREP TIME:** 12 minutes **COOK TIME:** 18 minutes
SERVES 4

Salmon turns out beautiful when roasted lightly caramelized and perfectly moist. Bok choy is packed with minerals, vitamins, and fiber. If you can't find bok choy, try halved Brussels sprouts prepared the same way.

4 (4-ounce) salmon fillets

Sea salt

Freshly ground black pepper

4 teaspoons olive oil, divided

¼ cup maple syrup

¼ cup sesame seeds

16 baby bok choy, quartered

Juice of 1 lemon

1. Preheat the oven to 400°F. Line a baking sheet with parchment paper and set aside.

2. Season the salmon with salt and pepper.

3. In a large skillet, heat 1 teaspoon of the oil over medium-high heat. Pan-sear the salmon on both sides for about 3 minutes in total, turning halfway through. Place the fish on one-third of the baking sheet. Spread maple syrup on each fillet and top with sesame seeds.

4. In a large bowl, toss the bok choy, remaining 3 teaspoons of oil, and lemon juice. Season with salt and pepper and spread on the remaining two-thirds of the baking sheet.

5. Bake until the fish flakes easily with a fork and the bok choy is tender-crisp, about 15 minutes. Serve.

Per Serving: Calories: 329; Total fat: 17g; Saturated fat: 3g; Sodium: 108mg; Carbohydrates: 19g; Sugar: 12g; Fiber: 5g; Protein: 25g

Caprese Fish and Bean Bake

DAIRY-FREE, GLUTEN-FREE **PREP TIME:** 10 minutes **COOK TIME:** 20 minutes **SERVES** 4

Caprese is an Italian salad with tomato, basil, mozzarella, and balsamic vinegar. This fish and bean casserole is inspired by those flavors. Tomato is a lovely low-calorie veggie high in inflammation-fighting lycopene. And the dark leafy green base is packed with antioxidants such as lutein and zeaxanthin. These will protect the eyes from cataracts and macular degeneration, which are common diabetes complications.

Nonstick
cooking spray

1 (15-ounce) can
low-sodium white
beans, drained
and rinsed

1 cup baby
spinach leaves

1 cup chopped
Swiss chard

12 medium
tomatoes, chopped

4 (4-ounce)
halibut fillets

Sea salt

Freshly ground
black pepper

2 teaspoons olive oil

1 tablespoon chopped
fresh basil

1. Preheat the oven to 400°F. Lightly coat a 10-inch square baking dish with cooking spray.

2. Layer the beans, spinach, Swiss chard, and tomatoes in the bottom of the baking dish. Place the fish in the baking dish, season with salt and pepper, and drizzle with the olive oil.

3. Cover with foil and bake for about 20 minutes, until the fish flakes easily.

4. Serve topped with basil.

Per Serving: Calories: 290; Total fat: 5g; Saturated fat: 1g; Sodium: 164mg; Carbohydrates: 33g; Sugar: 10g; Fiber: 9g; Protein: 31g

Fish Tacos with Avocado Salsa

|||||||||||||||||||||||||||||||||||||||||||||||||||||||||||||||||||||||||||||||||||||||||||||||||||

DAIRY-FREE, GLUTEN-FREE **PREP TIME:** 20 minutes **COOK TIME:** 10 minutes
SERVES 4

*Fish tacos are a staple dish in California, and are now a
healthy and delicious menu option all over North America.
The avocado salsa is a perfect creamy counterpart to the
delicate fish. Avocado is high in fiber and healthy fats, so it
does not raise blood sugar levels. The salsa can be made up
to 2 days ahead with lots of lime juice to prevent oxidation.*

**1 teaspoon
blackening spice**

**4 (4-ounce)
haddock fillets**

1 teaspoon olive oil

**1 avocado, pitted
and diced**

1 tomato, chopped

**1 scallion, both white
and green parts,
finely chopped**

**1 tablespoon chopped
fresh cilantro**

Juice of 1 lime

**8 (4-inch) corn
tortillas, at room
temperature**

**1 cup finely
shredded lettuce**

1. Rub the blackening spice all over the fish.

2. In a large skillet, heat the oil over
   medium-high heat. Pan-sear the fish for
   about 10 minutes in total, turning halfway through, until just cooked through
   and golden. Transfer the fish to a plate
   and, using a fork, break the fish into
   large chunks.

3. While the fish is cooking, in a large bowl,
   combine the avocado, tomato, scallion,
   cilantro, and lime juice.

4. Divide the fish among the tortillas and top
   with the salsa and lettuce. Fold the tortillas
   over and serve 2 per person.

Per Serving: Calories: 259; Total fat: 10g; Saturated fat: 1g;
Sodium: 252mg; Carbohydrates: 23g; Sugar: 2g; Fiber: 6g;
Protein: 22g

Salmon Po'boy

PREP TIME: 20 minutes **COOK TIME:** 10 minutes **SERVES** 4

The Po'boy sandwich is an institution in New Orleans. This lighter version uses salmon with creamy cabbage slaw on whole-wheat rolls. The carrot in the slaw adds a pretty flash of color, and this veggie is low sugar. Carrots are rich in beta-carotene, which can contribute to blood sugar control.

4 (4-ounce) skinless salmon fillets

2 teaspoons Cajun seasoning

2 teaspoons olive oil

1 cup finely shredded cabbage

1 large carrot, shredded

1 scallion, both white and green parts, sliced

¼ cup low-fat plain Greek yogurt

1 tablespoon apple cider vinegar

1 teaspoon maple syrup

4 crusty whole-wheat rolls, halved

1. Preheat the oven to 400°F.

2. Season the salmon fillets with the Cajun seasoning.

3. In a large ovenproof skillet, heat the oil over medium-high heat. Pan-sear the salmon for 2 minutes per side, then place the skillet in the oven. Roast for about 6 minutes, until just cooked through. Remove the salmon from the oven and set it aside.

4. While the salmon is cooking, in a large bowl, toss the cabbage, carrot, scallion, yogurt, vinegar, and maple syrup until well combined.

5. Place a salmon fillet on each roll and top with of the cabbage mixture. Serve.

Per Serving: Calories: 326; Total fat: 11g; Saturated fat: 3g; Sodium: 276mg; Carbohydrates: 25g; Sugar: 5g; Fiber: 3g; Protein: 30g

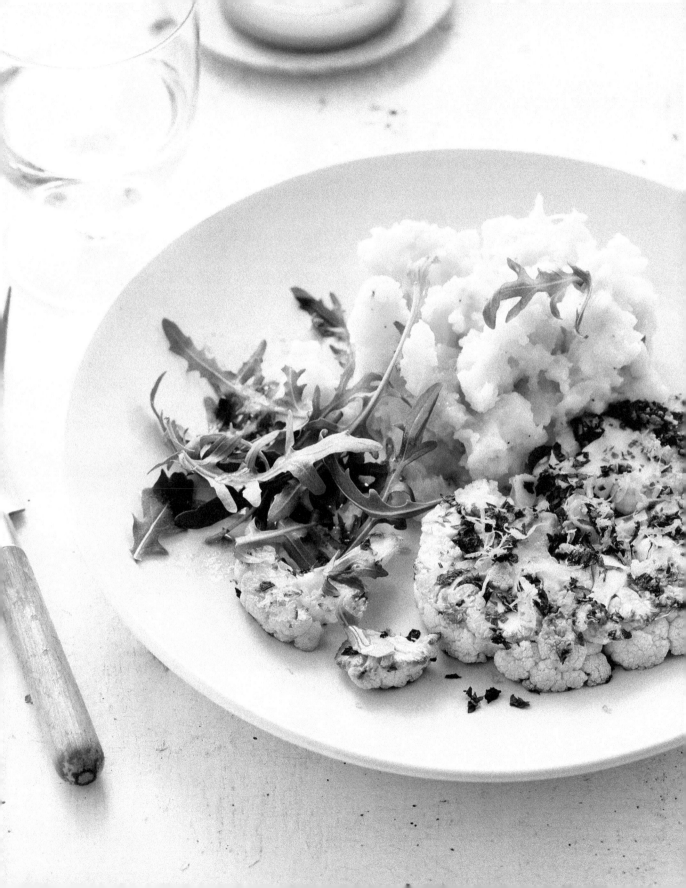

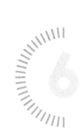

VEGETARIAN

Navy Bean Soup with Spinach

GLUTEN-FREE, VEGAN **PREP TIME:** 10 minutes **COOK TIME:** 20 minutes **SERVES** 2

If I were to open a restaurant, it would be soup themed; I love soup and make it at least once a week. This recipe is a stick-to-the-ribs meal packed with fiber-rich veggies and legumes in a flavorful broth. If you are freezing it, omit the spinach until you reheat the soup.

2 teaspoons olive oil

1 onion, chopped

2 celery stalks, diced

2 teaspoons minced garlic

3 cups sodium-free vegetable broth

1 (15-ounce) can low-sodium great northern beans, drained and rinsed

2 carrots, peeled and diced

1 tomato, diced

1 cup baby spinach

2 teaspoons chopped fresh thyme, or 1 teaspoon dried thyme

Sea salt

Freshly ground black pepper

1. In a medium stockpot, heat the oil over medium-high heat. Sauté the onion, celery, and garlic for about 5 minutes, until softened.

2. Add the broth, beans, carrots, and tomato and bring to a boil. Reduce the heat to low and simmer for about 13 minutes, until the carrots are tender. Add the spinach and thyme and simmer for an additional 2 minutes.

3. Season with salt and pepper and serve.

VARIATION: *Any type of legume works here. Try lentils, black beans, chickpeas, or split peas in the same amount as the great northern beans.*

Per Serving: Calories: 293; Total fat: 5g; Saturated fat: 1g; Sodium: 165mg; Carbohydrates: 50g; Sugar: 11g; Fiber: 15g; Protein: 14g

Tomato Vegetable Soup

GLUTEN-FREE, VEGAN **PREP TIME:** 10 minutes **COOK TIME:** 20 minutes **SERVES** 2

I make this soup in the summer when the produce is plentiful and seasonal, but it is delicious in any season. Try it with a sprinkle of grated Parmesan or feta cheese. This might remind you of minestrone, and you can add a can of cannellini beans to increase the similarity as well as the amount of fiber.

2 teaspoons olive oil

1 onion, chopped

2 celery stalks, chopped

1 red bell pepper, seeded and chopped

2 teaspoons minced garlic

3 cups low-sodium vegetable broth

1 (15-ounce) can no-salt-added diced tomatoes

1 carrot, peeled and chopped

1 cup small cauliflower florets

½ cup green beans, trimmed and cut into 1-inch pieces

Sea salt

Freshly ground black pepper

1. In a large stockpot, heat the oil over medium-high heat. Sauté the onion, celery, bell pepper, and garlic for about 5 minutes, until softened.

2. Add the broth, tomatoes and their juices, carrot, cauliflower, and green beans to the pot. Bring the soup to a boil, reduce the heat to low, and simmer for about 15 minutes, until the vegetables are crisp-tender.

3. Season with salt and pepper and serve.

Per Serving: Calories: 160; Total fat: 6g; Saturated fat: 1g; Sodium: 175mg; Carbohydrates: 26g; Sugar: 13g; Fiber: 10g; Protein: 5g

Red Lentil Dal with Pita

||||||||||||||||||||||||||||||||||||||||||||||||||||||||||||||||||||||||||||||||||||||||||||||||||||||||||||||||||||||||||

VEGAN **PREP TIME:** 10 minutes **COOK TIME:** 20 minutes **SERVES** 4

Traditional dal is made with yellow split peas, but lentils also break down nicely to create the requisite thick texture. Try hot curry paste or add a generous drizzle of chili oil if you enjoy a little heat. Dal is lovely served over rice and freezes beautifully for up to 1 month in a sealed container.

1 cup red lentils, rinsed

1 teaspoon olive oil

1 onion, finely chopped

1 teaspoon minced garlic

1 tablespoon mild curry paste

1 (15-ounce) can no-salt-added crushed tomatoes

Juice of ½ lemon

¼ cup chopped fresh cilantro

Whole-wheat pita bread or naan, for serving

1. In a medium saucepan, cover the lentils with 2-inches of water and bring to a boil over high heat. Boil until the lentils are tender, about 12 minutes. Drain and set aside.

2. While the lentils are cooking, in a large saucepan, heat the oil over medium-high heat. Sauté the onion and garlic for about 3 minutes, until softened.

3. Reduce the heat to medium-low and cook for about 5 minutes, until heated through and thick.

4. Top with cilantro and serve with pita or naan wedges.

PREP TIP: *Use 2 (15-ounce) cans drained lentils. Cook them until boken down, about 12 minutes.*

Per Serving: Calories: 293; Total fat: 3g; Saturated fat: 0g; Sodium: 141mg; Carbohydrates: 53g; Sugar: 4g; Fiber: 11g; Protein: 16g

Whole-Grain Pasta Primavera

VEGETARIAN **PREP TIME:** 10 minutes **COOK TIME:** 20 minutes **SERVES** 4

Primavera means "spring" in Italian, which makes sense when you see the heaps of tender vegetables in this dish. Use any veggie you have in your refrigerator; the ones here are just a guideline. Add a pinch or two of red pepper flakes if you like a bit of heat.

8 ounces whole-grain penne pasta

1 tablespoon olive oil

2 cups sliced mushrooms

½ onion, chopped

2 teaspoons minced garlic

2 cups broccoli florets

Juice and zest of 1 lemon

1 tablespoon chopped fresh basil, or 1 teaspoon dried basil

Freshly ground black pepper

¼ cup grated Parmesan cheese

1. Fill a large saucepan three-quarters full of water and bring it to a boil over high heat. Add the pasta and cook for about 20 minutes, until al dente.

2. While the pasta is cooking, in a large skillet, heat the oil over medium-high heat and sauté the mushrooms, onion, and garlic until browned, about 8 minutes.

3. When the pasta has 2 minutes left to cook, add the broccoli, lemon juice, lemon zest, and basil to the skillet and cook until the broccoli is tender-crisp, about 2 minutes.

4. Drain the pasta and add to the skillet, tossing to combine. Season with pepper and serve topped with Parmesan cheese.

MAKE-AHEAD: *Cook the pasta ahead and refrigerate in a sealed container for up to 3 days. Add it along with the broccoli and heat!*

Per Serving: Calories: 288; Total fat: 6g; Saturated fat: 2g; Sodium: 130mg; Carbohydrates: 50g; Sugar: 4g; Fiber: 7g; Protein: 13g

Broiled-Vegetable Sandwich

VEGETARIAN **PREP TIME:** 15 minutes **COOK TIME:** 7 minutes **SERVES** 2

I must admit I was not a fan of eggplant or zucchini—until I tasted these veggies broiled. They become sweeter and smoky tasting, and the texture transforms. Don't skip broiling the rolls—otherwise the juices from the vegetables can make them soggy.

½ eggplant, cut into ¼-inch slices

1 red bell pepper, seeded and cut into 1-inch strips

1 zucchini, cut lengthwise into ¼-inch strips

½ red onion, cut into ¼-inch slices

1 tablespoon olive oil

1 tablespoon balsamic vinegar

1 tablespoon chopped fresh oregano

Sea salt

Freshly ground black pepper

2 whole-wheat kaiser rolls, halved

¼ cup crumbled low-fat feta cheese

Handful baby spinach leaves

1. In a large bowl, toss the eggplant, bell pepper, zucchini, onion, oil, vinegar, oregano, salt, and pepper.

2. Preheat the oven to broil. Spread the veggies on a baking sheet.

3. Broil the vegetables until they are lightly charred and softened, turning once halfway through, about 6 minutes total. Transfer the vegetables to a plate.

4. Broil the buns, cut-side up, for about 1 minute. Top the bottom half the toasted buns with the broiled vegetables. Sprinkle with the feta cheese and spinach and top with the other half of the bun. Serve.

PREP TIP: *These veggies are also fabulous grilled. Cook them on medium-high heat for about the same time.*

Per Serving: Calories: 314; Total fat: 14g; Saturated fat: 4g; Sodium: 257mg; Carbohydrates: 40g; Sugar: 15g; Fiber: 10g; Protein: 11g

Asiago-Garlic Cauliflower Steaks

GLUTEN-FREE, VEGETARIAN **PREP TIME:** 10 minutes **COOK TIME:** 20 minutes
SERVES 2

I discovered cauliflower steaks was in a charming restaurant Guelph, Ontario, called the Babel Fish. I never considered cutting whole heads of fiber-rich cauliflower into thick slabs and cooking them like meat. You can top cauliflower with almost any sauce, herb, spice, or cheese to create wonderful variations.

Nonstick cooking spray

1 large cauliflower head, cut into 4 (1½-inch) thick steaks (base intact)

2 tablespoons olive oil

Juice and zest of 1 lemon

1 teaspoon minced garlic

½ teaspoon sea salt

Freshly ground black pepper

¼ cup shredded Asiago cheese

Chopped fresh parsley, for garnish

1. Preheat the oven to 400°F. Lightly cover a baking sheet with cooking spray.

2. In a small bowl, stir together the olive oil, lemon juice, lemon zest, garlic, and salt until blended.

3. Brush each cauliflower steak with the olive oil mixture and season with pepper.

4. Bake until golden brown, about 20 minutes, flipping halfway through.

5. Serve immediately, sprinkled with Asiago and parsley.

VARIATION: *Try cabbage instead of cauliflower. Remove the outer leaves and trim the woody stalk. Don't cut too much off, or the steaks will come apart.*

Per Serving: Calories: 301; Total fat: 18g; Saturated fat: 4g; Sodium: 421mg; Carbohydrates: 28g; Sugar: 9g; Fiber: 10g; Protein: 13g

Mediterranean Whole-Wheat Couscous

VEGETARIAN **PREP TIME:** 10 minutes, plus 10 minutes **COOK TIME:** 10 minutes **SERVES** 4

In North Africa, couscous is cooked in pots big enough for an adult to sit in comfortably. Couscous is not a grain; it is pasta made with semolina. This recipe uses whole-wheat couscous for its nutty, almost sweet taste and fiber content.

1 cup whole-wheat couscous

2 large tomatoes, chopped

1 yellow bell pepper, seeded and chopped

¼ red onion, chopped

10 Brussels sprouts, thinly sliced

2 tablespoons chopped fresh oregano

3 tablespoons extra-virgin olive oil

1 tablespoon balsamic vinegar

Sea salt

Freshly ground black pepper

2 tablespoons crumbled low-fat feta cheese

1. Place the couscous in a medium bowl and add 2 cups of boiling water. Cover and set aside for 10 minutes. Fluff with a fork and add the tomatoes, bell pepper, onion, Brussels sprouts, and oregano. Stir to combine.

2. In a small bowl, whisk together the olive oil and vinegar and add the dressing to the couscous mixture, tossing to mix well.

3. Season with salt and pepper and serve sprinkled with feta cheese.

MAKE-AHEAD: *The couscous can be made up to 3 days ahead and refrigerated. You can also use quinoa, bulgur, or wheat berries.*

Per Serving: Calories: 335; Total fat: 11g; Saturated fat: 2g; Sodium: 109mg; Carbohydrates: 49g; Sugar: 4g; Fiber: 6g; Protein: 10g

Asparagus and Cherry Tomato Zoodles

GLUTEN-FREE, VEGETARIAN **PREP TIME:** 20 minutes **SERVES** 2

This dish is gorgeous and is an ideal centerpiece for an alfresco meal on a sunny patio. The colors form the tomatoes and olives, and cheese look like a still-life painting. The delicious, earthy-tasting kale has over 30 percent of the daily recommended amount of fiber in this serving size.

2 tablespoons extra-virgin olive oil

1 tablespoon freshly squeezed lemon juice

1 teaspoon grainy mustard

1 teaspoon chopped fresh basil

⅛ teaspoon freshly ground black pepper

12 asparagus spears, trimmed, cut into ribbons with a vegetable peeler

20 cherry tomatoes, halved

2 cups chopped baby kale

¼ cup pitted kalamata olives, sliced

¼ cup crumbled low-fat goat cheese

1. In a small bowl, whisk together the olive oil, lemon juice, mustard, basil, and pepper, and set aside.

2. In a large bowl, toss the asparagus, tomatoes, kale, and olives until well mixed. Add the dressing and mix.

3. Top with goat cheese and serve.

PREP TIP: *If you have a mandoline slicer, you can use it to create the asparagus ribbons.*

Per Serving: Calories: 243; Total fat: 18g; Saturated fat: 4g; Sodium: 234mg; Carbohydrates: 17g; Sugar: 6g; Fiber: 8g; Protein: 8g

Falafel Pitas

VEGETARIAN **PREP TIME:** 17 minutes **COOK TIME:** 13 minutes **SERVES** 4

Falafel is a traditional Middle Eastern dish that is usually deep-fried and served in folded flatbread called taboon. *This recipe is baked to reduce the fat but retains all the lovely flavor. These tasty patties can be served alone, as a salad topping, or on a platter with dips as an appetizer.*

3 teaspoons olive oil, divided

½ onion, chopped

1 teaspoon minced garlic

1 (15-ounce) can low-sodium chickpeas, drained and rinsed

1 large egg

¼ cup whole-wheat bread crumbs or almond flour

1 teaspoon ground cumin

¼ teaspoon ground turmeric

Sea salt

1. In a small skillet, heat 1 teaspoon of the oil over medium-high heat and sauté the onion and garlic for about 3 minutes, until softened.

2. Transfer the onion mixture to a blender and add the chickpeas, egg, bread crumbs, cumin, and turmeric, and pulse until the mixture holds together when pressed. Season with salt and pepper.

3. Divide the mixture into 16 portions, roll them into balls, and flatten slightly. You can either refrigerate or cook them.

4. In a large skillet, heat the remaining 2 teaspoons of oil over medium heat. Cook the patties for about 10 minutes in total, turning once, until golden on both sides.

Freshly ground black pepper

4 (4-inch) whole-wheat pitas, halved

2 cups shredded lettuce

½ cup Tzatziki Sauce (page 127) or store-bought

5. Serve 2 falafels stuffed into each pita half, topped with shredded lettuce and tzatziki sauce.

Per Serving: Calories: 267; Total fat: 10g; Saturated fat: 2g; Sodium: 289mg; Carbohydrates: 35g; Sugar: 6g; Fiber: 8g; Protein: 12g

Tomato-Basil Flatbread Pizza

VEGETARIAN **PREP TIME:** 15 minutes **COOK TIME:** 5 minutes **SERVES** 4

When considering a treat meal, this is my husband's choice every time. Better than takeout, it features the classic flavor combination of tomato and basil with some extra vegetables for good measure. And since you pick the ingredients, the meal is healthier. I sometimes make this on the barbecue set to medium-low heat for a superb smoky finish.

1 (10- to 12-inch) whole-grain flatbread

¼ cup homemade or prepared sundried tomato or basil pesto

1 large tomato, chopped

½ cup chopped canned artichoke hearts

¼ cup chopped baby kale

¼ cup shredded reduced-fat mozzarella cheese

¼ cup roughly chopped fresh basil

1. Place a rack in the middle of the oven and preheat the oven to broil.

2. Place the flatbread on a baking sheet and spread the pesto all over it, leaving about ½ inch bare around the edges. Scatter the tomato, artichoke hearts, and kale all over the crust and top evenly with mozzarella.

3. Broil until the crust is crispy and the cheese is melted, about 5 minutes. Top with basil and serve.

VARIATION: *Pre-made whole-grain pizza crust is an excellent option here, and you can use your favorite toppings instead of the ones in this recipe.*

Per Serving: Calories: 256; Total fat: 10g; Saturated fat: 2g; Sodium: 374mg; Carbohydrates: 30g; Sugar: 3g; Fiber: 6g; Protein: 8g

Chickpea Curry

GLUTEN-FREE, VEGAN **PREP TIME:** 10 minutes **COOK TIME:** 20 minutes **SERVES** 4

When my mother came to North America, she made only three recipes, and curry was her best. This coconutty dish is inspired by the handful of unsweetened shredded coconut she tossed into the pot. You can serve this curry with a fresh green salad or whole-wheat naan bread instead of rice.

1 cup brown rice, soaked overnight in water and drained

1 tablespoon olive oil

1 onion, chopped

1 tablespoon minced garlic

1 (15-ounce) can low-sodium diced tomatoes

1 (15-ounce) can low-sodium chickpeas, drained and rinsed

½ cup light coconut milk

2 carrots, peeled and diced

1½ tablespoons curry powder

1 cup baby spinach leaves

1. Fill a large saucepan three-quarters full of water and bring to a boil over high heat. Add the drained rice, cover, reduce the heat to low, and simmer for about 20 minutes, until the rice is tender. Drain the excess water, cover, and set aside.

2. While the rice is simmering, in a large skillet, heat the oil over medium-high heat and sauté the onion and garlic for about 3 minutes, until softened.

3. Add the tomatoes and their juices, chickpeas, coconut milk, carrots, and curry powder, and bring to a boil. Reduce the heat to low and simmer for about 15 minutes, until the carrots are tender. Stir in the spinach and simmer for 2 minutes.

4. Serve over the rice.

Per Serving: Calories: 388; Total fat: 13g; Saturated fat: 6g; Sodium: 166mg; Carbohydrates: 60g; Sugar: 8g; Fiber: 11g; Protein: 10g

Summer Squash Feta Frittata

GLUTEN-FREE, VEGETARIAN **PREP TIME:** 10 minutes **COOK TIME:** 15 minutes **SERVES** 4

Frittata is a versatile Italian dish that is basically a crust-less quiche. You can add almost anything to it, even cooked whole-grain pasta. Eggs are a stellar source of protein, and you can purchase omega-3 eggs to boost your intake of that healthy fatty acid.

8 large eggs

½ cup skim milk or unsweetened non-dairy milk

2 teaspoons dried thyme

¼ teaspoon sea salt

⅛ teaspoon freshly ground black pepper

1 tablespoon olive oil

¼ onion, chopped

2 cups chopped zucchini or other summer squash

1. Preheat the oven to broil.

2. In a large bowl, whisk together the eggs, milk, thyme, salt, and pepper until well combined.

3. In a large ovenproof skillet, heat the oil over medium-high heat. Sauté the onion for about 3 minutes, until softened. Add the zucchini and sauté for about 3 minutes, until softened.

4. Add the egg mixture to the skillet and cook the frittata, lifting the edges of the cooked egg to allow the uncooked egg to flow underneath.

1 tomato, chopped

½ cup shredded low-fat Swiss cheese

5. When the frittata is just set, after about 8 minutes, remove from the heat and sprinkle the tomato and cheese on top.

6. Put the skillet in the oven and broil for about 1 minute, until the cheese is melted and the frittata is cooked through.

7. Cut into wedges and serve.

Per Serving: Calories: 227; Total fat: 13g; Saturated fat: 4g; Sodium: 296mg; Carbohydrates: 7g; Sugar: 5g; Fiber: 1g; Protein: 19g

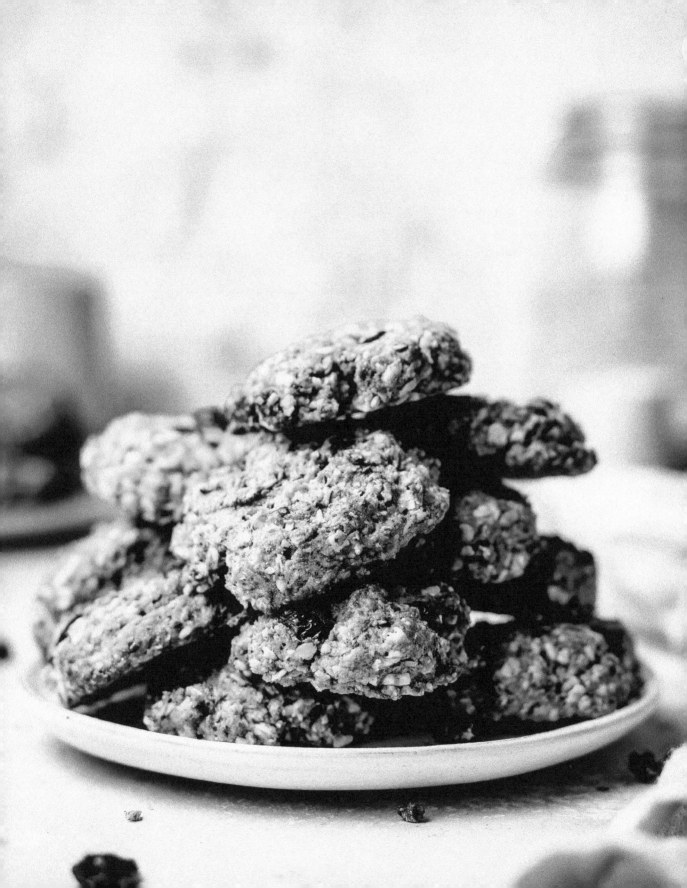

DESSERTS AND STAPLES

Pear and Pecan Crumble

GLUTEN-FREE, VEGETARIAN **PREP TIME:** 10 minutes **COOK TIME:** 20 minutes
SERVES 6

The scent of buttery fruit, toasty pecans, and warm spices will waft through your entire house as this lovely dessert bakes. The whole grains, pears, and flaxseed add a generous amount of healthy fiber to this dish. Flaxseed also contains a group of chemical compounds called lignans, which can stabilize glucose control.

2 teaspoons butter

4 pears, peeled, cored, and sliced

1 tablespoon cornstarch

½ teaspoon ground cinnamon

¼ teaspoon ground nutmeg

1 cup rolled oats

½ cup chopped pecans

¼ cup almond flour

2 tablespoons ground flaxseed

1. Preheat the oven to 400°F.

2. In a medium ovenproof skillet, melt the butter over medium heat and sauté the pears for about 5 minutes, until tender-crisp and purged of juices.

3. Stir in the cornstarch, cinnamon, and nutmeg and set aside.

4. In a medium bowl, toss the oats, pecans, almond flour, flaxseed, cinnamon, cloves, and salt until well mixed.

5. Add the melted butter and maple syrup and toss until the mixture resembles coarse crumbs.

½ teaspoon ground cinnamon

¼ teaspoon ground cloves

¼ teaspoon sea salt

¼ cup melted butter

2 tablespoons maple syrup

6. Top the fruit in the skillet evenly with the crumble mixture.

7. Put the skillet in the oven and bake for about 15 minutes, until golden. Serve warm.

MAKE-AHEAD: *The entire recipe can be put together and placed in the refrigerator for up to 3 days. Remove from the refrigerator and bake in the same heated oven for 25 minutes. You can also make the crumbles in 6-ounce ramekins and bake for 15 minutes.*

Per Serving: Calories: 348; Total fat: 18g; Saturated fat: 7g; Sodium: 171mg; Carbohydrates: 40g; Sugar: 15g; Fiber: 11g; Protein: 4g

Chocolate Yogurt Granita

GLUTEN-FREE, VEGETARIAN **PREP TIME:** 5 minutes, plus freezing time **SERVES** 4

Chocolate is an all-time favorite treat for many, and this simple dessert certainly satisfies any craving for it. Cocoa is very rich in inflammation-fighting antioxidants and is low on the glycemic index. For a truly decadent granita, add a table-spoon of peanut butter to the mixture.

2 cups low-fat plain Greek yogurt

½ cup unsweetened almond milk

¼ cup unsweetened cocoa powder

2 tablespoons maple syrup

2 teaspoons pure vanilla extract

1. Place the yogurt, almond milk, cocoa powder, maple syrup, and vanilla in a blender and blend until very smooth.

2. Pour the mixture into a metal 9-inch square baking dish and place in the freezer. Stir with a fork every 30 minutes or so for about 3 hours, until frozen and the mixture resembles soft snow. Serve.

PREP TIP: *You can also use an ice cream maker if you have one available. Just follow the manufacturer's instructions.*

Per Serving: Calories: 134; Total fat: 3g; Saturated fat: 2g; Sodium: 93mg; Carbohydrates: 19g; Sugar: 14g; Fiber: 3g; Protein: 8g

Vanilla Bean N'Ice Cream

GLUTEN-FREE, VEGAN **PREP TIME:** 5 minutes **SERVES** 4

When you blend frozen bananas, they turn into a luscious dessert with a soft-serve ice cream consistency. Although sweet, bananas still rank as a low glycemic index food and can be enjoyed in moderation. For different variations, add sugar-free chocolate chips, peanut butter, chopped strawberries, or even a teaspoon of espresso powder for a healthy sweet treat.

3 overripe bananas, cut into chunks and frozen

¼ cup unsweetened vanilla almond milk

1 vanilla bean, seeds scraped out

Pinch salt

1. Place the bananas, almond milk, vanilla bean, and salt in a blender and blend until it is a soft-serve texture.

2. Serve immediately or freeze in a sealed container for up to 2 weeks. Let the n'ice cream sit at room temperature for about 10 minutes before scooping.

VARIATION: *You can use 2 teaspoons of pure vanilla extract instead of vanilla bean.*

Per Serving: Calories: 83; Total fat: 0g; Saturated fat: 0g; Sodium: 47mg; Carbohydrates: 20g; Sugar: 10g; Fiber: 3g; Protein: 1g

Apple Pie Parfait

GLUTEN-FREE, VEGETARIAN **PREP TIME:** 25 minutes **SERVES** 2

Don't be fooled by this list of very humble ingredients; they are a scrumptious treat when combined. Yogurt adds protein, and the apple and almonds provide heart-friendly fiber. Almonds are rich in magnesium, which can improve insulin sensitivity, so add a few more if you like the extra crunch.

1 apple, peeled, cored, and chopped

1 teaspoon maple syrup (optional)

½ teaspoon ground cinnamon

1 cup low-fat vanilla yogurt, divided

¼ cup chopped almonds or pecans, divided

¼ cup whipped coconut cream (see tip)

1. In a small bowl, toss together the apple, maple syrup (if using), and cinnamon until well mixed.

2. Layer ¼ cup yogurt in the bottom of a tall, wide glass or small bowl. Then layer in ¼ of the apple and 1 tablespoon almonds. Repeat the layering and top the glass with 2 tablespoons of whipped coconut cream.

3. Repeat with a second glass or bowl and serve immediately.

PREP TIP: *To make whipped coconut cream, take a chilled can of coconut milk and scoop off the top solid section into a medium bowl. Whip with electric hand beaters or a whisk until fluffy. You can add a dash of maple syrup if you want the cream a little sweeter, but it is delicious without.*

Per Serving: Calories: 311; Total fat: 20g; Saturated fat: 11g; Sodium: 87mg; Carbohydrates: 23g; Sugar: 15g; Fiber: 4g; Protein: 9g

Oatmeal-Cranberry Cookies

VEGETARIAN **PREP TIME:** 15 minutes **COOK TIME:** 10 minutes **MAKES** 18 cookies

Quinoa is a strange ingredient for cookies, but it adds tenderness and a pleasing nutty taste. Since quinoa is a complete protein—containing all essential amino acids—it helps with the uptake of the carbs in these treats. This means your blood sugar levels remain stable.

½ cup melted butter

¼ cup honey

1 large egg

1 teaspoon pure vanilla extract

1 cup white whole-wheat flour

1 cup rolled oats

1 cup leftover cooked quinoa

½ cup dried cranberries

½ teaspoon baking soda

¼ teaspoon baking powder

¼ teaspoon ground nutmeg

¼ teaspoon sea salt

⅛ teaspoon ground allspice

1. Preheat the oven to 375°F. Line a baking sheet with parchment paper.

2. In a large bowl, mix the butter, honey, egg, and vanilla.

3. In a medium bowl, stir the flour, oats, quinoa, cranberries, baking soda, baking powder, nutmeg, salt, and allspice until well combined.

4. Add the dry ingredients to the wet ingredients and stir until combined.

5. Scoop the batter in heaped tablespoons onto the baking sheet and flatten out.

6. Bake for 10 minutes, or until golden brown.

7. Store the cookies in a sealed container at room temperature for 5 days or freeze for up to 1 month.

Per Serving (1 cookie): Calories: 127; Total fat: 6g; Saturated fat: 3g; Sodium: 98mg; Carbohydrates: 16g; Sugar: 6g; Fiber: 2g; Protein: 2g

Everyday Balsamic Vinaigrette

||||||||||||||||||||||||||||||||||||||||||||||||||||||||||||||||||||||||||||||||||||||||||||||||||||

GLUTEN-FREE, VEGAN **PREP TIME:** 10 minutes **MAKES** about ¾ cup

Dressings are the best place to use a quality extra-virgin olive oil because the clean flavor shines through. Olive oil is high in monounsaturated fat, which can help lower "bad" LDL cholesterol and support a healthy cardiovascular system. If you prefer, you can use another type of vinegar, such as apple cider or even plain distilled.

½ cup extra-virgin olive oil

¼ cup balsamic vinegar

2 teaspoons chopped fresh oregano

1 teaspoon Dijon mustard

1 teaspoon chopped fresh thyme

Sea salt

Freshly ground black pepper

1. In a small bowl, whisk together the oil, vinegar, oregano, mustard, and thyme until well blended.

2. Season the dressing with salt and pepper. Store in a sealed container at room temperature for up to 1 week.

Per Serving (2 tablespoons): Calories: 170; Total fat: 18g; Saturated fat: 2g; Sodium: 38mg; Carbohydrates: 2g; Sugar: 2g; Fiber: 0g; Protein: 0g

Tzatziki Sauce

GLUTEN-FREE, VEGETARIAN **PREP TIME:** 15 minutes **MAKES** 1½ cups

The first tzatziki I made was in Tripoli with homemade yogurt and cucumbers and dill I grew myself. It was delicious and felt like a real accomplishment, and you can also make your own at home with little effort. Make sure you use Greek yogurt instead of regular because it contains more protein and fewer carbs.

1 cup low-fat plain Greek yogurt

½ English cucumber, grated, with all the liquid squeezed out

Juice of ½ lemon

1 tablespoon chopped fresh dill

1 teaspoon minced garlic

Sea salt

Freshly ground black pepper

1. In a small bowl, stir together the yogurt, cucumber, lemon juice, dill, and garlic until well blended.

2. Season with salt and pepper. Refrigerate the sauce in a sealed container for up to 5 days.

Per Serving (¼ cup): Calories: 31; Total fat: 1g; Saturated fat: 0g; Sodium: 55mg; Carbohydrates: 4g; Sugar: 3g; Fiber: 1g; Protein: 2g

Smoky Barbecue Sauce

GLUTEN-FREE, VEGAN **PREP TIME:** 10 minutes **COOK TIME:** 10 minutes
MAKES 1½ cups

Barbecue sauce is a tricky condiment for people with type 2 diabetes because store-bought and some homemade recipes are extremely high in sugar. This version doesn't compromise on flavor but is ideal for proteins such as chicken or steak or as a delicious spread for roasted-vegetable sandwiches. Try adding a half teaspoon of liquid smoke for even more flavor.

1 (15-ounce) can no-salt-added crushed tomatoes

2 tablespoons no-salt-added tomato paste

2 tablespoons apple cider vinegar

1 tablespoon smoked paprika

2 teaspoons garlic powder

1 teaspoon onion powder

Pinch ground cayenne pepper

1. In a medium saucepan, place the tomatoes, tomato paste, vinegar, paprika, garlic powder, onion powder, and cayenne over medium-low heat. Bring to a simmer, reduce the heat to low, and simmer for 10 minutes.

2. Let the sauce cool and refrigerate in a sealed container for up to 1 week.

Per Serving (2 tablespoons): Calories: 28; Total fat: 0g; Saturated fat: 0g; Sodium: 15mg; Carbohydrates: 6g; Sugar: 3g; Fiber: 1g; Protein: 1g

Basil Marinara Sauce

GLUTEN-FREE, VEGAN **PREP TIME:** 5 minutes **COOK TIME:** 25 minutes **SERVES** 6

Store-bought pasta sauce can be very high in salt and sugar, and those labeled "healthy" often have no flavor at all. This homemade creation is redolent with whole foods: garlic, onion, and a generous amount of basil and oregano. Try this sauce with your favorite whole-grain pasta, spiralized veggies, or shirataki noodles.

1 tablespoon olive oil

1 onion, chopped

1 tablespoon minced garlic

2 (28-ounce) cans no-salt-added crushed tomatoes

1½ tablespoons dried basil

2 teaspoons dried oregano

½ teaspoon sea salt

½ teaspoon freshly ground black pepper

Pinch red pepper flakes

1. In a large saucepan, heat the oil over medium-high heat. Sauté the onion and garlic for about 3 minutes, until softened.

2. Stir in the tomatoes, basil, oregano, salt, pepper, and red pepper flakes, and bring to a boil. Reduce the heat to low, partially cover, and simmer for 20 to 25 minutes.

3. Adjust the seasonings, cool, and refrigerate in a sealed container for up to 1 week or freeze for up to 3 months.

Per Serving: Calories: 75; Total fat: 3g; Saturated fat: 0g; Sodium: 124mg; Carbohydrates: 12g; Sugar: 8g; Fiber: 6g; Protein: 3g

Quick Pickles

GLUTEN-FREE, VEGAN **PREP TIME:** 10 minutes, plus chilling time

COOK TIME: 2 minutes **SERVES** 6

Pickles can be high in sodium, but the vinegary brine may help lower blood sugar levels by improving the body's response to insulin. Homemade pickles are also healthier—you can control the salt level. Make your pickles fancier by storing them in mason jars with a couple sprigs of fresh dill.

1 cup white vinegar

2 garlic cloves, crushed

1 tablespoon granulated sugar

1½ teaspoons mustard seed

1½ teaspoons dried dill

1 teaspoon sea salt

1 bay leaf

8 small (Kirby, if possible) cucumbers, cut into 1-inch slices

1. In a medium saucepan, combine the vinegar, garlic, sugar, mustard seed, dill, salt, and bay leaf over medium-high heat. Bring the mixture to a simmer, stirring To dissolve the sugar, for about 2 minutes.

2. Place the cucumbers in a large bowl and pour the vinegar mixture over them, stirring to coat. Cool them to room temperature, and then refrigerate until chilled.

3. Remove the bay leaf and serve. Refrigerate the pickles in a sealed container for up to 1 week.

VARIATION: *Try other vegetables such as cauliflower florets, jalapeño peppers, pearl onions, and sliced carrots along with the cucumbers.*

Per Serving: Calories: 34; Total fat: 0g; Saturated fat: 0g; Sodium: 56mg; Carbohydrates: 8g; Sugar: 3g; Fiber: 1g; Protein: 1g

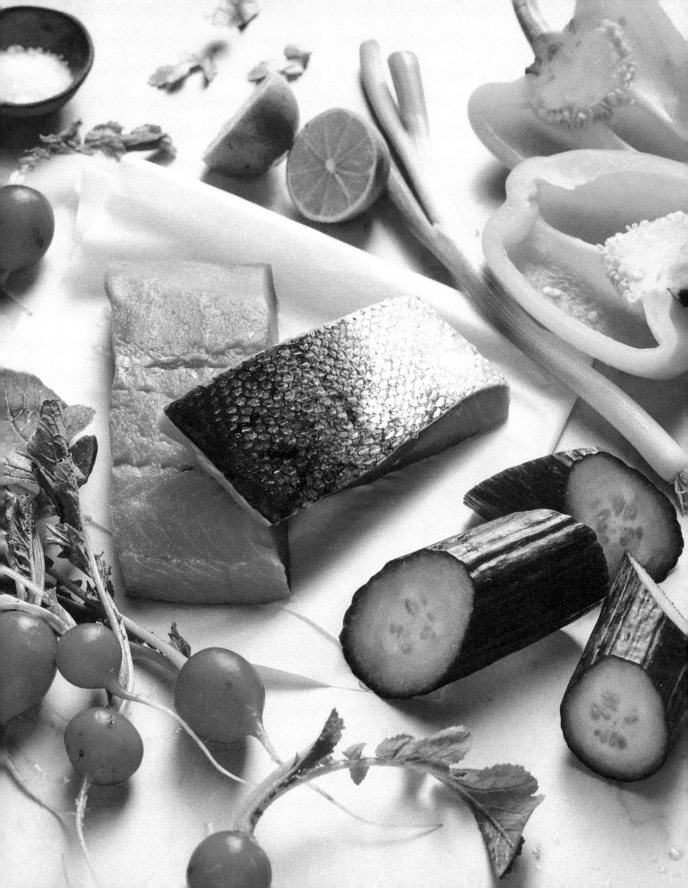

Measurement Conversions

Volume Equivalents	U.S. Standard	U.S. Standard (ounces)	Metric (approximate)
Liquid	2 tablespoons	1 fl. oz.	30 mL
	¼ cup	2 fl. oz.	60 mL
	½ cup	4 fl. oz.	120 mL
	1 cup	8 fl. oz.	240 mL
	1½ cups	12 fl. oz.	355 mL
	2 cups or 1 pint	16 fl. oz.	475 mL
	4 cups or 1 quart	32 fl. oz.	1 L
	1 gallon	128 fl. oz.	4 L
Dry	⅛ teaspoon	—	0.5 mL
	¼ teaspoon	—	1 mL
	½ teaspoon	—	2 mL
	¾ teaspoon	—	4 mL
	1 teaspoon	—	5 mL
	1 tablespoon	—	15 mL
	¼ cup	—	59 mL
	⅓ cup	—	79 mL
	½ cup	—	118 mL
	⅔ cup	—	156 mL
	¾ cup	—	177 mL
	1 cup	—	235 mL
	2 cups or 1 pint	—	475 mL
	3 cups	—	700 mL
	4 cups or 1 quart	—	1 L
	½ gallon	—	2 L
	1 gallon	—	4 L

Oven Temperatures

Fahrenheit	Celsius (approximate)
250°F	120°C
300°F	150°C
325°F	165°C
350°F	180°C
375°F	190°C
400°F	200°C
425°F	220°C
450°F	230°C

Weight Equivalents

U.S. Standard	Metric (approximate)
½ ounce	15 g
1 ounce	30 g
2 ounces	60 g
4 ounces	115 g
8 ounces	225 g
12 ounces	340 g
16 ounces or 1 pound	455 g

References

American Diabetes Association. "6. Glycemic Targets: *Standards of Medical Care in Diabetes—2021." Diabetes Care* 44, supplement 1 (January 2021): S73–S84. doi.org/10.2337/dc21-S006.

Becerra-Tomás, Nerea, Andrés Díaz-López, Nuria Rosique-Esteban, Emilio Ros, Pilar Buil-Cosiales, Dolores Corella, Ramon Estruch, et al. "Legume Consumption Is Inversely Associated with Type 2 Diabetes Incidence in Adults: A Prospective Assessment From the PREDIMED Study." *Clinical Nutrition* 37, no. 3 (June 2018): 906–913. doi.org/10.1016/j.clnu.2017.03.015.

Centers for Disease Control and Prevention. "National Diabetes Statistics Report, 2020." CDC.gov/diabetes/data/statistics-report/index.html.

Christensen, Allan S., Lone Viggers, Kjeld Hasselström, and Soren Gregersen. "Effect of Fruit Restriction on Glycemic Control in Patients with Type 2 Diabetes—A Randomized Trial." *Nutrition Journal* 12, no. 29 (March 5, 2013). doi.org/10.1186/1475-2891-12-29.

Hegde, Shreelaxmi V., Prabha Adhikari, Nandini M, and Vivian D'Souza. "Effect of Daily Supplementation of Fruits on Oxidative Stress Indices and Glycaemic Status in Type 2 Diabetes Mellitus." *Complementary Therapies in Clinical Practice* 19, no. 2 (May 2013): 97–100. doi.org/10.1016/j.ctcp.2012.12.002.

Johnson, Evan C., Costas N. Bardis, Lisa T. Jansen, J.D. Adams, Tracie W. Kirkland, and Stavros A. Kavouras. "Reduced Water Intake Deteriorates Glucose Regulation in Patients with Type 2 Diabetes." *Nutrition Research* 43 (July 2017): 25–32. doi.org/10.1016/j.nutres.2017.05.004.

Jovanovski, Elena, Rana Khayyat, Andreea Zurbau, Allison Komishon, Nourah Mazhar, John L. Sievenpiper, Sonia Blanco Mejia, et al. "Should Viscous Fiber Supplements Be Considered in Diabetes Control? Results From a Systematic Review and Meta-analysis of Randomized Controlled Trials." *Diabetes Care* 42, no. 5 (May 2019): 755–766. doi.org/10.2337/dc18-1126.

Ramdath, D., Simone Renwick, and Alison M. Duncan. "The Role of Pulses in the Dietary Management of Diabetes." *Canadian Journal of Diabetes* 40, no. 4 (August 2016): 355–363. doi.org/10.1016/j.jcjd.2016.05.015. PMID: 27497151.

Saito, Yuuki, Shizuo Kajiyama, Ayasa Nitta, Takashi Miyawaki, Shinya Matsumoto, Neiko Ozasa, Shintaro Kajiyama, et al. "Eating Fast Has a Significant Impact on Glycemic Excursion in Healthy Women: Randomized Controlled Cross-Over Trial." *Nutrients* 12, no. 9 (September 10, 2020): 2767. doi.org/10.3390/nu12092767.

Takahashi, Keiko, Chiemi Kamada, Hidenori Yoshimura, Ryota Okumura, Satoshi Iimuro, Yasuo Ohashi, Atsushi Araki, et al. "Effects of Total and Green Vegetable Intakes on Glycated Hemoglobin A1C and Triglycerides in Elderly Patients with Type 2 Diabetes Mellitus: The Japanese Elderly Intervention Trial." *Geriatrics & Gerontology International* 12, supplement 1 (April 2012): 50–58. doi.org/10.1111/j.1447-0594.2011.00812.x.

United States Department of Agriculture. "Food Availability and Consumption." Last modified August 25, 2021. ERS.USDA.gov/data-products/ag-and-food-statistics-charting-the-essentials/food-availability-and-consumption/.

van Son, Jenny, Ivan Nyklíček, Victor J. Pop, Marion C. Blonk, Ronald J. Erdtsieck, Pieter F. Spooren, Arno W. Toorians, et al. "The Effects of a Mindfulness-Based Intervention on Emotional Distress,

Quality of Life, and HbA (1C) in Outpatients With Diabetes (DiaMind): A Randomized Controlled Trial." *Diabetes Care* 36, no. 4 (April 2013): 823–830. doi.org/10.2337/dc12-1477.

Viguiliouk, Effie, Cyril W.C. Kendall, Sonia Blanco Mejia, Adrian I. Cozma, Vanessa Ha, Arash Mirrahimi, Viranda H. Jayalath, et al. "Effect of tree nuts on glycemic control in diabetes: a systematic review and meta-analysis of randomized controlled dietary trials." *PLoS One* 9, no. 7 (July 30, 2014): e103376. doi.org/10.1371/journal .pone.0103376.

Viguiliouk, Effie, Sarah E. Stewart, Viranda H. Jayalath, Alena Praneet Ng, Arash Mirrahimi, Russell J. de Souza, Anthony J. Hanley, et al. "Effect of Replacing Animal Protein with Plant Protein on Glycemic Control in Diabetes: A Systematic Review and Meta-analysis of Randomized Controlled Trials." *Nutrients* 7, no. 12 (December 1, 2015): 9804–9824. doi.org/10.3390/nu7125509.

Willett, Walter, JoAnn Manson, and Simin Liu. "Glycemic Index, Glycemic Load, and Risk of Type 2 Diabetes." *The American Journal of Clinical Nutrition* 76, no. 1 (July 1, 2002): 274S–280S. doi.org/10.1093/ajcn/76.1.274S.

Index

About the Authors

Andy De Santis

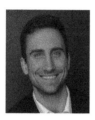

Andy is a private practice dietitian, blogger, and multi-time published author from Toronto, Canada. He has written for a wide of array of print and online publications both locally and for platforms across the globe. Andy graduated from the University of Toronto Dalla Lana School of Public Health in 2014 with a master's degree in public health nutrition before starting his career at Diabetes Canada, where he worked in the research and education department and fostered his passion for nutrition communication. He went on from there to pursue a multi-year journey as a health writer and private practice dietitian, having extensively studied and applied much of the nutrition science he shares in this book along the way.

Michelle Anderson

Michelle Anderson is the author and certified ghostwriter of over 50 cookbooks focused on healthy diets and delicious food. She worked as a professional chef for over 25 years, honing her craft overseas in North Africa and all over Ontario, Canada, in fine-dining restaurants. She worked as a corporate executive chef for RATIONAL Canada for four years, collaborating with her international counterparts and consulting in kitchens all over southern Ontario and in the United States. Her focus is food as medicine and using field to fork wholesome quality ingredients in vibrant visually impactful dishes. Michelle lives in Temiskaming Shores, Ontario, Canada, with her husband, two sons, two Newfoundland dogs, and three cats.